Client-Centred Practice in Occupational Therapy

Dedication

To Marjorie and Clarence for all they taught me about love and my rural roots
To Juri for his faith in me and for teaching me that life is to be lived
To Doe whose creative example gave me the courage to go it alone
And to all my friends who believed in me when I never could.

For Churchill Livingstone:

Editorial Director: Mary Law
Project Development Manager: Valerie Dearing
Project Manager: Jane Shanks

Client-Centred Practice in Occupational Therapy

A Guide to Implementation

Edited by

Thelma Sumsion
Lecturer and Course Leader, MScOT Programme, Brunel University, London, UK

Forewords by

Christine Craik
Director of Undergraduate Occupational Therapy, Brunel University, London, and former Chair of the College of Occupational Therapists

John Glossop
Chairman of Lancaster Disablement Information and Support Centre

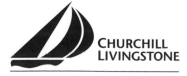

CHURCHILL LIVINGSTONE

EDINBURGH LONDON NEW YORK PHILADELPHIA SYDNEY TORONTO

CHURCHILL LIVINGSTONE
An imprint of Harcourt Brace and Company Limited

© Harcourt Brace and Company Limited 1999

is a registered trademark of Harcourt Brace and
Company Limited

The right of Thelma Sumsion to be identified as editor of
this work has been asserted by her in accordance with the
Copyright, Designs and Patents Act 1988

First published 1999

ISBN 0 443 06127 0

British Library Cataloguing in Publication Data
A catalogue record for this book is available from the British
Library

Library of Congress Cataloging in Publication Data
A catalog record for this book is available from the Library
of Congress

Note
Medical knowledge is constantly changing. As new information becomes available, changes in treatment, procedures, equipment and the use of drugs become necessary.
The contributors and the publishers have, as far as it is
possible, taken care to ensure that the information given in
this text is accurate and up-to-date. However, readers are
strongly advised to confirm that the information, especially
with regard to drug usage, complies with the latest
legislation and standards of practice.

The
publisher's
policy is to use
**paper manufactured
from sustainable forests**

Printed in China

Contents

Contributors

Anne Carswell PhD OT(C)
Associate Professor and Director, School of
Rehabilitation Science, University of British
Columbia, Vancouver, British Columbia, Canada
*Anne is one of the authors of the Canadian
Occupational Performance Measure (COPM).*

Marie Gage MSc BSc(OT) OT(C)
Collective Wisdom Management, Haliburton,
Ontario, Canada
*Marie teaches client-centred care planning to
interdisciplinary care teams that are interested in
integrating their care.*

Sandra Jean Graham Hobson MAEd OT(C)
Associate Professor, School of Occupational
Therapy, University of Western Ontario,
London, Ontario, Canada
*Sandra teaches client-centred practice in relation to
older adults with cognitive impairment and young
adults with acquired brain injury.*

Alice Kusznir MEd OT(C)
Occupational Therapist-in-chief and Senior
Occupational Therapist – Mood and Anxiety
Program, Centre for Addictions and Mental
Health, Toronto, Ontario, Canada
*Alice has been working with persons with
mental health disabilities for 20 years and has
a particular interest in mood disorders as well
as client-centred practice.*

Mary Ann McColl PhD OT(C)
Head, Occupational Therapy Division, and
Professor, School of Rehabilitation Therapy,
Queen's University, Kingston, Ontario, Canada
*Mary Ann is one of the authors of the Canadian
Occupational Performance Measure (COPM).*

Davina Parker MSc Dip COT SROT
Occupational Therapy Manager, University
Hospital Birmingham NHS Trust, Birmingham,
UK
*Davina carried out her dissertation on the Canadian
Occupational Performance Measure and has
implemented client-centred practice within an acute
hospital, a hospice and a rehabilitation unit.*

Nancy Pollock MSc OT(C)
Associate Clinical Professor, School of
Rehabilitation Science, McMaster University,
Hamilton, Ontario, Canada
*Nancy is one of the authors of the Canadian
Occupational Performance Measure (COPM).*

Elizabeth Scott MSc OT(C)
Administrative Director, Society Women and
Health Program, Centre for Addictions and
Mental Health – Clarke Division and Assistant
Professor, Department of Occupational Therapy,
University of Toronto, Toronto, Ontario, Canada
*Elizabeth has been exploring issues related to
client-centred practice for several years, particularly
in relation to mental health and quality of health.*

Thelma Sumsion MEd BSc (OT) SROT
Lecturer and Course Leader, MScOT
Programme, Brunel University, London, UK
*Thelma has been interested in client-centred practice
since the early 1980s when she chaired the Canadian
taskforce that created the Occupational Therapy
Guidelines for Client Centred Practice.*

Forewords

The concept of client-centred practice has been afforded greater or lesser recognition at different times during the history of occupational therapy, but it is clearly at the heart of the profession. At some points in the past, occupational therapists have had to struggle against the restrictions of the medical model to uphold the philosophy of client-centred practice. The terms used to describe this way of working have also altered and will probably continue to do so, reflecting changes in terminology rather than changes in philosophy.

Whatever it is named, the essence of occupational therapy is the collaboration or partnership between the client and the therapist, working together to achieve the client's goals. Although this philosophy is central to occupational therapy, understanding its true meaning and putting it into practice have always been more difficult than most occupational therapists acknowledge.

This timely book brings together, in a clear and logical way, the philosophy of client-centred practice, the academic underpinning that contributes to its development and, probably of most importance for therapists, the practical application of the philosophy. The editor has assembled a distinguished group of authors with the knowledge and credentials to help us to understand the concepts and implement them. The book has many case studies which illustrate client-centred practice in a meaningful way. Having read the poignant story of Nick in Chapter 6, who could deny the justification for providing the red wheelchair?

Most occupational therapists today would claim to work within a client-centred model; however, few of us would be able to demonstrate this effectively. This book will help us to produce the evidence to achieve this effective implementation. There has seldom been a more auspicious time for client-centred practice. Guided by this book, occupational therapists now have the opportunity to practise what we have always believed.

1999   Christine Craik

I am an ex-teacher and in 1983 I was disabled by a sub-arachnoid haemorrhage. I am a wheelchair user and a partially sighted hemiplegic. I am married, have three children, a dog, a cat and two goldfish.

I am unique, I am not a collection of symptoms and physical problems, I am more than the sum of my disabilities. My goals may not be your goals; things which you consider necessary to your very existence may be of little or no importance to me.

Before my brain haemorrhage I sailed competitively. An outdoor pursuits centre went to great efforts to arrange for me to sail in a trimaran specially adapted for the disabled. It took hours to rig the boat and winch me aboard. Sailing must incorporate some degree of danger or adrenalin rush but this was safe to the point of boredom and I have never sailed since.

I have to live with my disabilities 24 hours a day; I am disabled at weekends, on bank holidays and even on Christmas Day. Crises do not occur to suit professionals. Also, I am not a saint! I do things which I know are bad for me and enjoy doing them. I am lazy and therapies are more likely to be effective when incorporated into my lifestyle. The therapeutic use of a heavy beer glass should not be ignored and my coordination has been greatly improved by the repetitive action of filling and lighting my pipe, though the close proximity of a fire extinguisher is advisable.

I am a member of a family and their needs must be taken into consideration. A bathroom full of ironwork is fine as long as there's room for teenage daughters, who spend half a lifetime in there with face packs and hair dye; don't offer me a single bed no matter how medically sound. I am a husband and father who happens to be disabled.

I am on the Course Committee of the Occupational Therapy Degree Course at St Martin's College, Lancaster and was involved with the validation of the Course. I had the pleasure of meeting Thelma Sumsion whilst speaking at an OT conference and found that we had many ideas in common.

I am a strong proponent of client-centred practice and hope that in future this common sense approach crosses into other disciplines.

1999   John Glossop

Preface

My interest in client-centred practice began in the early 1980s when I chaired the first in a series of working groups organised by the Canadian Association of Occupational Therapists (CAOT). This work continued for many years and resulted in several publications, many of which are discussed in this text, designed to educate occupational therapists about and assist them with the implementation of client-centred practice. The members of these groups were inspirational and both therapists and clients owe a great deal to their commitment to client-centred practice.

Since the early 1980s Canadian therapists have struggled with many challenges related to the implementation of client-centred practice, and research published in professional journals addresses many of these issues. This text aims to continue the development of this area of practice by combining information about the theoretical and practical aspects of client-centred practice.

The contributing authors were chosen because of their interest in and knowledge of client-centred practice as well as their varied expertise in working with a range of client groups.

I moved to England in 1996 and quickly became aware of the interest therapists throughout the UK shared with their Canadian colleagues. They too were struggling with the concepts of client-centred practice and the most effective ways of implementing this approach. This awareness gave birth to the idea for this book and the invitation to authors from both Canada and England to share their expertise. It is my hope that therapists in several countries will find helpful information in this book that will remove the barriers to the implementation of client-centred practice and strengthen their commitment to this approach for the benefit of their clients.

1999   Thelma Sumsion

1

Overview of client-centred practice

T. Sumsion

This chapter presents the core concepts of client-centred practice that must be clearly understood before successful implementation is achieved. A variety of models and definitions is discussed with a focus on the Canadian Model of Occupational Performance (CMOP). Clinical examples are provided in the discussion of the components of the CMOP, and the relationship of this approach to other approaches used by occupational therapists is briefly outlined.

EMERGING IMPORTANCE OF CLIENT-CENTRED PRACTICE

Client-centred practice is emerging as an important approach to intervention in all areas of occupational therapy. The reasons for this emergence are complex and are based on the realisation that the client is the most important component of any intervention. In the daily work of a therapist it often seems that the budget, the current approach to management or staff shortages prevail and dictate how work is performed. However, inclinations to succumb to these forces must be overcome and a balance achieved that places the client firmly in the position of receiving the full potential of all the therapist's abilities.

Health promotion, which emerged as an important concept within health care in the 1980s, laid the foundation for clients to be involved in health care and to be responsible for their own health. Health promotion, as defined by the World Health Organisation, is 'the process of enabling people to increase control over and to improve their health, (WHO 1984). The recognition of the importance of these concepts has facilitated their integration into many programmes that fully support consumer awareness. Further developments in the 1990s have seen the emergence of consumer-led and self-help groups which strive to meet needs outside the realm of professional involvement. These are truly client-centred programmes. Consumer rights, human rights and the technological revolution have also hastened the development of client-centred practice (Gage 1994, Law et al 1995).

Therapists should also be aware that the College of Occupational Therapists supports the client-centred approach to intervention by stating within the Code of Ethics and Professional Conduct that services should be client centred and needs led. This document also reminds therapists that 'each client is unique and brings an individual perspective to the occupational therapy process' (College of Occupational Therapists 1995). It is important that therapists understand the implications of these statements and have the necessary information to implement this approach.

Many government and organisation initiatives have also ingrained the right of clients to make decisions about the course of intervention and to assume responsibility for their own health care. The Patient's Charter, published by the Department of Health in 1995, is an example of a document that supports the principles of client-centred practice. The term 'client centred' does not appear within the charter but the principles underlying this approach are well ingrained in the wording. These principles include the right to make choices, to have all necessary information before a decision is made and to have access to necessary services (Department of Health 1995).

Universities are also acknowledging the need to change the way future therapists and doctors are educated. The medical school at a major Canadian university has recently adopted a patient-centred method as the focus of the curriculum. This method recognises that the patient has a disease but also an illness experience that is unique to that individual. The student-centred programme introduces a case at the beginning of each week. Students interview the patient, discuss issues and spend the week learning what they need to know to treat the patient (Western Alumni 1997). Throughout this process the focus is on the patient, not the therapist.

The above examples might lead to the conclusion that client-centred practice is fully supported by all health professionals. However, as will be outlined in this book, there are many aspects of this approach that provide a considerable challenge to the fundamental beliefs of many therapists. There continues to be a struggle among health professionals concerning the conflict that arises between the client's role in decision-making and the values of the patient and the professional (Emmanuel & Emmanuel 1992). A client-centred approach certainly places new demands on all those involved (Wilson 1985).

All of these issues provided the impetus for this book, which attempts to facilitate the implementation of client-centred practice. It has been written for all therapists whether they work as clinicians, managers, educators or consultants, or are in the process of training to be clinicians. The information is also relevant to therapists in all work settings including hospitals, communities, schools, universities and industries. The focus is both theoretical and practical with an emphasis on providing solutions to some of the more challenging aspects of implementation.

The book begins with an overview of a variety of models of client-centred practice with a focus on the Canadian Model of Occupational Performance, which was designed by occupational therapists. Subsequent chapters address the client-centred approach, environmental considerations and implementation issues. A manager provides detailed information about how to implement a client-centred approach within a department. The next series of chapters addresses implementation issues with specific client groups including those with cognitive impairments, the elderly and clients with mental health and physical problems. The final chapter provides information about the Canadian Occupational Performance Measure, which is an appropriate outcome measure to conclude the discussion. All the contributing authors believe in client-centred practice and share the wish that 'client centered will be more than the latest catch phrase' (Sherr Klein 1997).

This is a book about client-centred practice and therefore client is the preferred term when referring to the person or persons with whom the occupational therapist interacts. In subsequent chapters the term client is used consistently. However, in this chapter the term patient is used occasionally if that was the term preferred by the authors whose work is being discussed. Both male and female pronouns are used to refer to clients and therapists throughout this book with no preference to either sex intended.

MODELS OF CLIENT-CENTRED PRACTICE

Client-centred practice is not unique to occupational therapy. Several models that focus on the client have been proposed by other disciplines. Robinson's model (1991) shows a patient-centred environment that integrates patient care needs into the design and delivery of all services. The model has three major components. The first is organisational self-care which refers to the organisation's concern with the need for support and care for its health-care providers. The second component, partners in health care, acknowledges the interdependent roles of health-care providers and the need for communication and collaboration among all players. The final aspect is masters of change. In today's environment change is inevitable and continuous, and there are many dynamics that accompany that change and which providers must be prepared to address. Any model that hopes to improve services for clients must also address the needs of the providers.

Levenstein et al (1986) focus on the potential for patients and doctors to have different agendas. The doctor's agenda is to assign a differential diagnosis through history-taking, physical examination and laboratory investigation. The patient brings expectations, feelings and fears, and seeks to understand the illness experience. In a patient-centred approach the doctor's aim is to ascertain the patient's agenda

and to reconcile this with his or her own. This reconciliation leads to integration and a positive outcome for both the client and the physician.

Integration is facilitated through the consideration of the six interacting components of the patient-centred process (Stewart et al 1995). These components are:

- exploring both the disease and the illness experience
- understanding the whole person
- finding common ground regarding management
- incorporating prevention and health promotion
- enhancing the patient–doctor relationship
- being realistic.

Each of these components can be broken down into several aspects. For example, the illness experience includes the patient's ideas, feelings and the effect of the illness on function. The process of finding common ground focuses on problems, goals and the role of both the patient and the doctor. To enhance the patient–doctor relationship, issues such as the sharing of power and self-awareness must be considered (Stewart et al 1995). The final component focuses on being realistic. These two words require careful consideration as a major challenge of client-centred practice is working with the client to establish realistic goals. Little has been accomplished if the client emerges from the process with unrealistic goals that will impede progress rather than enhance it.

Speechley (1992) outlines a model from the Royal Marsden Hospital which stresses the partnership that needs to be created between the patient and the health professional. The professional brings an expert knowledge base and, hopefully, long-term support. The patient brings the experience of a chronic disease that is long term. Together these players can implement the plan of care and continue to re-evaluate it. This concept of partnership will receive further attention in several sections of this book.

These models all stress the important contributions that both the client and the practitioner bring to the intervention and the strength that results when these contributions are appropriately combined. These models also stress that the application of a client-centred approach is not simple as there are many things that must be learned and considered to ensure success. Perhaps a client-centred approach is just another way of thinking and a different attitude (Fehrsen & Henbest 1993). Asking oneself the following four questions will help to keep everything in perspective. Who am I talking to? Where is he from? What is his situation? And what is his problem? Weston et al (1989) expand on these questions by proposing several dimensions of the illness experience that physicians should explore. These dimensions are the patients' ideas, feelings and fears about what is wrong, their expectations of the doctor and the effect of illness on their functioning. All of these issues are relevant for occupational therapists attempting to understand occupational performance from the perspective of the client. Subsequent chapters of this book address a wide range of issues that will facilitate both the understanding and the application of client-centred practice.

DEFINITIONS

Before implementing client-centred practice it is important that the clinician has a clear definition of this approach. It is impossible to evaluate the effectiveness of an approach unless there is a clear definition of what has been applied. Many authors have discussed components of definitions related to patient-centred care and others have offered thoughtful complete definitions. One key feature of the patient-centred method is for the clinician to try to enter the patient's world and to see the illness through the patient's eyes (Brown et al 1989). McCracken et al (1983) elaborate on this concept by stating that the 'essence of the patient centered method is the physician's attempt to understand the meaning of the illness for the patient. Instead of, or as well as, interpreting the illness in terms of his own world the doctor tries to enter the patient's world. This involves answering the question, why did the patient come and what are his feelings, expectations and fears?' Henbest and Fehrsen (1992) also

support this approach. For these authors 'patient centred' means putting the person of the patient at the centre of the consultation and attempting to understand the patient's thoughts, feelings and expectations as well as his or her symptoms.

Other components of being patient centred include (Grol et al 1990):

- taking the patient and his or her problems, ideas and expectations seriously
- involving the patient in decisions
- giving information to enable patients to take responsibility for their own health
- feeling responsible for non-medical aspects of the presented problem.

Patient-centred care has been defined as 'individual and holistic care dictated by the needs and wishes of each patient'. The convenience of health-care professionals takes second place (Nuffield Institute 1995). A further definition states that the client-centred approach is 'based on the belief that the client is the important person in the relationship and that he has the resources and ability to help himself given the opportunity to do so' (Dexter & Walsh 1986).

There are few existing definitions of client-centred practice within occupational therapy. It is difficult to attempt to or succeed in applying anything that is not clearly defined or understood. The lack of a clear definition of client-centred practice and hence a clear guide for implementation has hindered the advancement of client-centred practice in occupational therapy (Gage 1994, McColl & Pranger 1994). In 1995 Law et al addressed this concern by defining client-centred practice as:

an approach to providing occupational therapy which embraces a philosophy of respect for and partnership with people receiving services. It recognises the autonomy of individuals, the need for client choice in making decisions about occupational needs, the strength clients 0bring to an occupational therapy encounter and the benefits of client–therapist partnership and the need to ensure that services are accessible and fit the context in which a client lives.

This definition focuses on many of the components presented in the Model of Occupational Performance, which is discussed in more detail below. This definition also adds several important concepts that the therapist brings to the encounter. These concepts include respect for the client and the partnership with the client. The client's autonomy, strength and need for choice must also be respected by the therapist. Issues related to the work environment such as the accessibility of services are also added for our consideration. However, it must be acknowledged that the therapist, client and the environment may also bring barriers to the implementation of client-centred practice. These barriers receive further attention in Chapters 4 and 9.

A research project in the UK in 1997 has created a draft of a British occupational therapy definition of client-centred practice. The first phase of this project used the Delphi Technique and enabled 63 therapists to participate in the creation of the definition. A series of four questionnaires was sent to these therapists over a period of several months. The first questionnaire outlined several aspects of client-centred practice from the literature and asked participants whether or not they agreed that these components should be included in the definition. They were asked to eliminate items that should not be included and to add additional components that they thought should be included. The second questionnaire provided therapists with the composite list of items from the first round. They were asked to prioritise five items from each of three sections that should be included in the definition. The three sections related to the therapist, the client and client-centred practice in general. The next questionnaire provided the results of this ranking and asked whether the participants agreed with the resulting five items in each section. These items were then used to create the draft definition which was sent to participants for final comment. The resulting draft definition (Sumsion 1999) is:

Client centred occupational therapy is a partnership between the therapist and client. The client's occupational goals are given priority and are at the centre of assessment and treatment. The therapist listens to and respects the client's standards and adapts the intervention to meet the client's needs. The client actively participates in negotiating goals for intervention and is empowered to make decisions

through training and education. The therapist and client work together to address the issues presented by a variety of environments to enable the client to fulfil his/her role expectations.

This project exemplifies the complexity of creating a relevant definition within a profession as diverse as occupational therapy. Wide consultation is required to ensure that as many factors as possible are considered. Therefore, this definition will be further refined in subsequent research projects that involve several additional groups of therapists. However, this draft presently serves as a working definition to guide the implementation of client-centred practice.

CLIENT-CENTRED PROGRAMMES

A therapist considering the implementation of a client-centred approach is advised to review examples of existing programmes presented by a range of disciplines. This review will highlight issues to be considered and facilitate learning based on the experiences of others. Fortunately there are many examples of programmes that have been designed from a client-centred perspective. A sample of these programmes is presented here and the reader is encouraged to read the references for more detailed information. Programmes focus on clients facing a wide range of problems and challenges. Wilson and Hobbs (1995) describe their client-centred programme, designed by a psychotic disorders team, as a therapeutic partnership. The focus is on alliance, accompaniment, agreement, action and accessibility. Consumer input is also important in programmes that occur at times of great emotional stress such as bereavement (Richmond et al 1994). Another aspect of client-centred programmes is limiting the number of intrusions into the client's home. Haig et al (1994) describe patient-oriented rehabilitation planning, which is comprehensive planning for people with limited access to services. They developed an evaluation tool called the quick programme. A previsit database is prepared and all team members complete specific assessments. This preplanning allows the rehabilitation plan to be agreed in a single visit. Client-centred programmes can also be offered in the hospital environment. One very innovative programme reserves half of the beds for a patient's family member or friend who acts as the patient's care partner during the hospital stay (Koska 1990).

The occupational therapy literature refers to the application of client-centred principles to a range of programmes from paediatrics to adult clients with cognitive impairment (Hobson 1996, Stewart & Harvey 1990). It is the contention of this book that client-centred practice can be used with any client group and in any setting, recognising that some client groups and settings pose greater challenges than others. Several issues to consider when applying client-centred practice to a range of clients are presented in subsequent chapters, which have been written by both British and Canadian therapists. In Chapter 6 Sandra Hobson addresses the complex issues related to applying a client-centred approach to work with clients with cognitive impairments. In Chapter 7 she discusses the equally challenging considerations when working with the elderly. In Chapter 8 Alice Kusznir and Elizabeth Scott present several case scenarios as examples of issues that arise when working with clients with mental health problems. Chapter 9 is the final one dedicated to a particular client group. In this chapter Marie Gage discusses the use of an interactive planning process with clients with physical disabilities. All of these discussions were written to assist therapists with the challenging realities of implementing client-centred practice.

OUTCOMES AND EVALUATION

The effectiveness of client-centred practice continues to be evaluated and many tools are emerging to help with this process. Chapter 10 discusses the Canadian Occupational Performance Measure (COPM), an outcome measure based on the principles of client-centred practice. Clinicians face many pressures that may limit the reality of using a client-centred approach unless it can be proven to be effective. Greenfield et al (1985) conducted a controlled study in which they encouraged patients to read their medical records, ask questions and negotiate decisions about their care. Despite poorer health the patients in the experimental group reported better role and physical functioning after the intervention than did the controls. Other authors have investigated the effectiveness of client-centred practice in other cultures and found support for the effectiveness of patient-centred interviewing (Henbest & Fehrsen 1992). Patient-centred consultations have been associated with improved patient outcomes including satisfaction and compliance, reduction of concern, symptom reduction and physiological status (Henbest & Stewart 1990, Stewart et al 1989). These few studies do not prove conclusively that a client-centred approach makes a difference to client well-being. However, they do provide sufficient evidence to support the continuation of studies in this area and to encourage therapists to continue to strive toward the effective implementation of client-centred practice.

MODEL OF OCCUPATIONAL PERFORMANCE

Occupational therapists are in the enviable position of having their own model on which to base client-centred interventions. The Model of Occupational Performance forms the basis of client-centred practice in occupational therapy. A Canadian Taskforce, funded jointly by the Canadian Association of Occupational Therapists (CAOT) and the Department of National Health and Welfare, developed this model. The model was presented in 1982 and was revised in 1983 and again in 1997. The original model was based on the work of Reed and Sanderson (1980) and places the individual in the centre of many interacting spheres (Fig. 1.1). The middle sphere depicts the three areas of a person's occupational performance, which are the focus of occupational therapy intervention. These areas are self-care, productivity and leisure. The performance components of the individual are featured in the centre sphere. These components are spiritual, physical, sociocultural and mental. Performance components are what make a person unique and what must be considered when discussing the areas of occupational performance. 'The essence

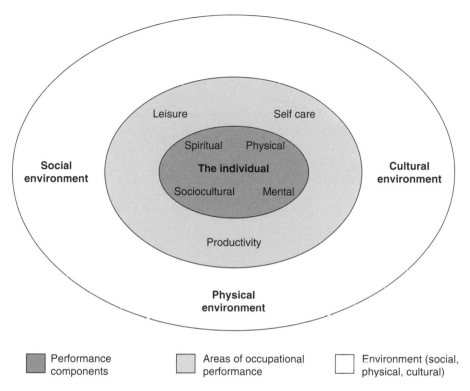

Figure 1.1 Interacting elements of the individual in a Model of Occupational Performance. (From Occupational therapy guidelines for client centred practice, Health Canada. Reproduced with permission of the Minister of Public Works and Government Services, Canada, 1997)

of a healthy functioning person is the balanced integration of these four performance components to provide a sense of well being' (Sumsion 1997). A client engages in the areas of occupational performance within a variety of environments. The original model focused on the social, physical and cultural environments, and in 1993 the political, economic and legal environments were added (CAOT 1993) (Fig. 1.2). In summary, this model suggests that there are many factors that influence a person's performance and which must be considered if the client-centred approach is to be implemented successfully (Sumsion 1993).

The name of the model was changed in 1997 to the Canadian Model of Occupational Performance (CMOP) (Fig. 1.3). This version of the model presents many new concepts. CMOP is a social model which places the person in a social–environmental context rather than locating the environment outside the person. The

new presentation also recognised the need to reconfigure the elements so the model appeared less static. It is now an interactive model showing relationships between persons, environment and occupation (L. Townsend, personal communication 1997). In reality therapists know that the interaction between the person, their roles and the environment is quite dynamic and must constantly accommodate a variety of changes. The new model allows for change and focuses on the interaction of the elements.

Self-care, productivity and leisure remain in the middle sphere but are now considered to be the key components of occupation. The central sphere now focuses on the person, with spirituality at the core and affective, cognitive and physical components also featured. The environments included in the outer sphere are physical, institutional, cultural and social (CAOT 1997). Each of these components will subsequently be discussed in more detail.

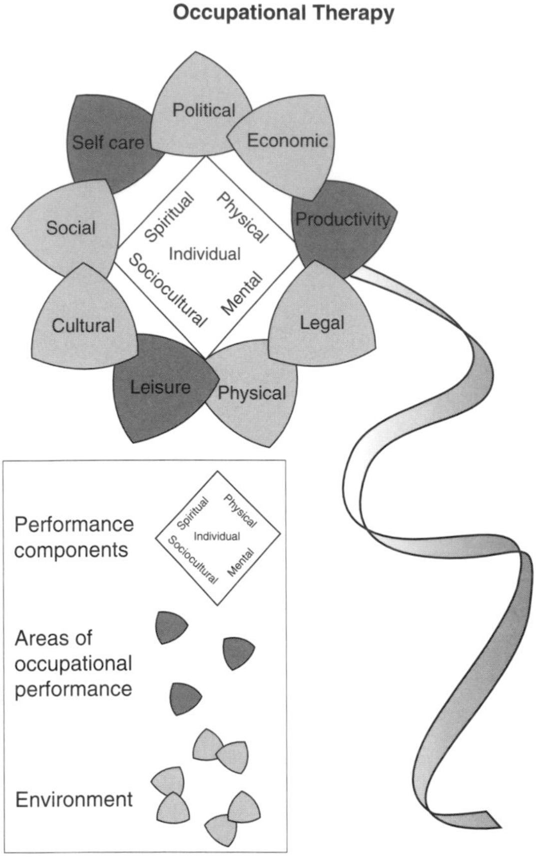

Occupational Therapy

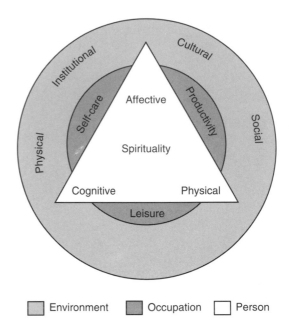

Figure 1.2 Interacting elements of the individual in a revised Model of Occupational Performance. (From Occupational therapy guidelines for client centred mental health practice, Health Canada. Reproduced with permission of the Minister of Public Works and Government Services, Canada, 1997)

This client-centred model can be applied to clients across the age span and in both institutional and community programmes. Before deciding whether this approach is appropriate, the therapist must consider how it can be applied in all stages of the occupational therapy process from the point of entry to the moment of discharge. This process is discussed further in Chapter 2.

Components of the model

A brief discussion of the components of occupation and the performance components of the Model of Occupational Performance is presented here as background to the subsequent chapters,

Figure 1.3 Canadian Model of Occupational Performance. (Reproduced with kind permission from Canadian Association of Occupational Therapists 1997 Enabling occupation: an occupational therapy perspective. CAOT Publications ACE, Ottawa, p. 32)

which facilitate the application of client-centred practice with a variety of adult populations. Issues from both the original and revised models are presented to enable therapists to find the combination that suits their approach to practice. Also, the Canadian Occupational Performance Measure (described in Chapter 10) and the study guide that accompanies it are based on the original model, which necessitates a clear understanding of its components. Many factors will determine where the emphasis of the intervention is placed but in order to make that decision a therapist must clearly understand the meaning of each component. A therapist must also understand that to work in a client-centred way is to ensure that all of these components are addressed.

Components of occupation

The components of occupation are self-care, productivity and leisure. Self-care originally referred to those activities or tasks that are done routinely to maintain the person's health and well-being in the environment (Reed & Sanderson 1980). The most recent document from the Canadian Association of Occupational Therapists presents a simpler definition of self-care as 'occupations for looking after the self' (CAOT 1997). Self-care involves more than personal grooming. For example, a client who has recently been confined to a wheelchair as a result of an industrial accident has to learn about the time factors necessary to accommodate a change in routine. She also has to consider necessary changes to the environment to accommodate her new form of mobility as well as how to organize, or perhaps reorganize, the performance of personal responsibilities such as childcare.

The second component is productivity, which was originally defined as 'those activities or tasks that are done to enable the person to provide support to the self, family and society through the production of goods and services' (Department of National Health and Welfare & Canadian Physiotherapy Association 1980). In the 1997 edition of the CMOP, productivity is defined as 'occupations that make a social or economic contribution or that provide for economic sustenance' (CAOT 1997). Productivity is not just paid employment. It involves whatever a person does to feel productive including paid or voluntary activities at home or in the community. Consider the case of a single woman who has worked all of her adult life as a nursing assistant and who is suddenly made redundant at age 56. It is highly unlikely that she will find paid employment when the number of unemployed people is so large. The challenge is to find activities that engage her and help her feel productive.

Leisure originally included the components of life that are free from work and self-care activities (CAOT 1991). However, leisure is now simply defined as occupations for enjoyment (CAOT 1997). This definition concerns various areas of focus for occupational therapists. Clients may need assistance in learning how to pursue familiar leisure activities in new ways as a result of injury or illness. A recently retired person who has always been too busy for leisure may wish to learn new activities. Someone who is depressed may want to learn to socialise in order to acquire the supports needed to cope with recurring episodes.

Performance components

Table 1.1 provides the definitions of the four original performance components as they appeared in the 1991 version of the Model of Occupational Performance. The 1997 document of the Canadian Association of Occupational Therapists has reformulated these performance components. The table shows the development of the original four components – mental, physical, spiritual and sociocultural – which could potentially be viewed in isolation from each other, into three components – affective, physical and cognitive – that facilitate interaction. These performance components have been defined individually in the table but they are all interdependent.

Occupational therapists are familiar with the affective, physical and cognitive performance components and regularly consider these in both assessment and treatment. However, the spiritual component is the most challenging one for therapists to incorporate into their practice. Its position has evolved from being one of the performance components, to being at the core of the Canadian Model of Occupational Performance. This new position is evidence of its importance. Christiansen (1997) supports the importance of spirituality by stating that 'if occupational therapy is to be complete and genuine in its consideration of humans as occupational beings, it must acknowledge spirituality as an important dimension of everyday life'.

Spirituality is in reality a part of all of the components of the model. 'It resides in persons, is shaped by the environment and gives meaning to occupation' (CAOT 1997). Several authors have addressed this concept within the occupational therapy literature, and recent editions of both the American and Canadian Journals of Occupational Therapy have been dedicated to a discussion of this performance component. Many authors have attempted to facilitate understanding and application of what can be challenging, personal concepts. Spirituality has

Table 1.1   Performance components

Performance components 1991	Performance components 1997
Mental – total emotional and intellectual response of an individual to the environment	Affective – (feeling) the domain that comprises all social and emotional functions and includes both interpersonal and intrapersonal factors
Physical – motor skills and sensory functions	Physical – (doing) the domain that comprises all sensory, motor and sensorimotor functions
Spiritual – state of well-being; the force that permeates and gives meaning to all life	
Sociocultural – dimension that describes the interpersonal relationships of a client with his or her family, and educational, ethnic and community backgrounds	
	Cognitive – (thinking) the domain that comprises all mental functions both cognitive and intellectual, and includes, among other things, perception, concentration, memory, comprehension, judgement and reasoning

Source: Canadian Association of Occupational Therapists 1991, 1997

been defined as an experience of meaning in everyday life. It is the true essence of the person and is connected to self, others and the rest of creation (Urbanowski & Vargo 1994). Spirituality can also be considered as the dignity and worth of the individual (Egan & Delaat 1994). Spirituality is, of course, an important component of religion, but these are not interchangeable terms. Spiritual matters are very personal, are linked to values and are also affected by cultural heritage. No one is suggesting that an occupational therapist should be able to address all of a client's spiritual needs. But it is important for a therapist to recognise that opportunities must be presented to clients for the expression of related issues and that success will be difficult to achieve without an understanding of this aspect of the client. All that may be necessary is for the therapist to listen closely to the client's expressed needs and to convey hope and acceptance. Occupational therapists will understand that this is a skilful application of one's self as a therapist (Egan & Delaat 1994, Urbanowski & Vargo 1994).

Therapists should be concerned about the inner strength that allows clients to keep functioning in the face of great challenges and adversity. Discussion of these issues is occurring at the national level. At a recent oncology workshop therapists discussed spirituality as a need for meaning and recognised that emptiness can occur with illness (Behan 1997). The acknowledgement of a spiritual dimension also encompasses the client's beliefs about power, control and the meaning of life (Christiansen 1997). How does a person with a high-level spinal lesion find the courage to tackle the challenges of everyday living? How does a parent with a severely disabled infant face all of the tomorrows of that child's life? How does a mother with terminal cancer stay strong when she knows she will not see her daughter graduate from college or marry? Surely the answer to these questions lies in the person's inner strength or their own interpretation of spirituality. Therefore the therapist has a role in helping the client to find that strength in a way that is meaningful to the client.

Environments

Information about the environments that were originally considered within two versions of the Model of Occupational Performance and the Canadian Model of Occupational Performance is presented briefly in Table 1.2. These environments are discussed more fully in Chapter 3. The original Model of Occupational Performance considered the cultural, physical and social environments and their impact on the client. A subsequent revision to the document mentioned the importance of also considering the legal, political and economic environments but did not define these terms. The inclusion of these three additional environments is an interesting statement about the development or decline of health care and the increasing prominence of legal and political issues. The latest version of the model has maintained the cultural, physical and social environments, and has encompassed the economic, legal and political environments within the institutional environment. It is important to remember that people are dynamically linked to a range of environments that will all impact on the challenges faced by clients as well as on the potential solutions to those challenges.

RELATIONSHIP OF THE MODEL OF OCCUPATIONAL PERFORMANCE TO OTHER APPROACHES

The increasing emphasis on evidence-based practice is rekindling the importance of establishing interventions based on proven models. This necessitates the study and review of relevant models and the choice of one or a combination of several as the basis of intervention. Client-centred practice is an approach that can readily be combined with other approaches to practice or other models. A client-centred approach ensures that the therapist and client work together as partners, that the client makes choices based on full information, and that the client is autonomous and has access to services. Therapists may choose to

Table 1.2 Environments

Environments 1991	Environments 1997
Cultural – ethos and value system of a particular people or group	Cultural – ethnic, racial, ceremonial and routine practices, based on ethos and value system of particular groups
Physical – natural and artificially made surroundings of an individual and structural living-space boundaries	Physical – natural and built surroundings that consist of buildings, roads, gardens, vehicles for transportation, technology, weather and other materials
Social – patterns of relationships of people living in an organised community	Social – social priorities about all elements of the environment, patterns of relationships of people living in an organised community, social groupings based on common interests, values, attitudes and beliefs
Legal*	Institutional – societal institutions and practices including policies, decision-making processes, procedures, accessibility and other organisational practices. Includes economic components … legal components … and political components
Political*	
Economic*	

Source: Canadian Association of Occupational Therapists 1991, 1993, 1997
* Canadian Association of Occupational Therapists 1993 (environments added to model but not defined)

use one or a variety of approaches to enhance and maximise the potential of this partnership. For example, the cognitive approach focuses on emotions, memory, attention, concentration, problem-solving, perception and creative thinking, which can all be connected to the performance components of the CMOP. Within this approach clients set their own goals and are taught coping skills, which are also central to a client-centred approach. The rehabilitative approach is compensatory and focuses on areas such as environmental adaptations. The CMOP provides detailed information about a range of environments that will enhance considerations relevant to these adaptations. This approach is flexible and responds to individual needs, and the individual is actively consulted and involved – key elements of a client-centred approach. Both of these approaches contain elements that work in harmony with client-centred practice. Both place at least some emphasis on response to individual priorities within the context of the challenges presented by both the client's problems and the relevant environment.

No attempt has been made to present a complete picture of all of the approaches with which occupational therapists work nor to enter the debate concerning the differences between a model, frame of reference or approach. However, the point has hopefully been made that client-centred practice works in harmony with many other approaches to practice. Things that are core to client-centred practice, such as clients setting their own goals, the therapist being flexible enough to ensure that the approach suits the client and providing the necessary education, are also key components of other approaches. The exception to this harmony may be the neurodevelopmental approach, which is prescriptive and allows little client choice, although the decision to use this approach could be reached in a client-centred way. Therapists should choose the model of practice that suits the environment in which they work and their own knowledge and skill, and then combine it with a client-centred approach.

Another issue that should be addressed before this introductory chapter is closed is whether or not it is possible to be partially client centred. Every qualified therapist knows that the greatest challenge is to find the right approach, which is as effective as possible for a particular client, and to apply that approach at the right time and in the right way. It is the combination of these elements that will enhance a successful outcome. In this regard client-centred practice is no different from any other approach. The skill in its successful application is to find the right combination that the client wants and can accept and that will enhance both short- and long-term goal attainment. Therefore it would appear that it is possible to be partially client centred if the appropriate components are applied to the individual's situation based on the client's goals and the issues presented by the relevant environments.

CONCLUSION

Occupational therapy is based on a holistic view of the client. Client-centred practice simply provides the formula and framework to ensure that occupational therapy is truly holistic and unique to each client. Practising from a client-centred perspective is more challenging than using the traditional prescriptive approach. The client and therapist work together to achieve the goals set by the client. The therapist is a facilitator who works in partnership with the client. Together they determine how the goals can be achieved in the context of all the relevant environments. The client makes the decisions based on the complete information that has been represented in an understandable format. There are barriers to the implementation of this approach but the strength of the partnership between the therapist and the client can overcome most obstacles. The level of therapist involvement will be determined by the client, but all clients can make some level of choice and deserve the opportunity to make all of the choices (Baum & Law 1997). The application of client-centred practice presents many challenges. Subsequent chapters provide the views of several therapists on how to address these concerns in a variety of clinical areas. Differing views have been encouraged to enable readers to choose a way to be client centred that fits with their chosen approach to intervention and the environmental pressures of their workplace.

REFERENCES

Baum C M, Law M 1997 Occupational therapy practice: focussing on occupational performance. American Journal of Occupational Therapy 51(4):277–288

Behan S 1997 The spiritual challenges of health care. Occupational Therapy News November:19

Brown J B, Weston W W, Stewart M A 1989 Patient centred interviewing. Part II: Finding common ground. Canadian Family Physician 35:153–157

Canadian Association of Occupational Therapists 1991 Occupational therapy guidelines for client centred practice. CAOT Publications ACE, Toronto

Canadian Association of Occupational Therapists 1993 Occupational therapy guidelines for client centred mental health practice. CAOT Publications ACE, Toronto

Canadian Association of Occupational Therapists 1997 Enabling occupation: an occupational therapy perspective. CAOT Publications ACE, Ottawa

Christiansen C 1997 Acknowledging a spiritual dimension in occupational therapy practice. American Journal of Occupational Therapy 51(3):169–172

College of Occupational Therapists 1995 Code of ethics and professional conduct for occupational therapists. College of Occupational Therapists, London

Delbanco T, Muller R, Chapman E 1990 Patient centred care: can your hospital afford not to have it? Hospitals November:48–54

Department of Health 1995 The patient's charter and you. DOH, London

Department of National Health and Welfare and the Canadian Physiotherapy Association 1980 Task force report: Toward assessment of quality of care in physiotherapy. DNHW–CPA, Ottawa

Dexter G, Walsh M 1986 Psychiatric nursing skills: a patient-centred approach. Croom Helm, Beckenham

Egan M, Delaat M D 1994 Considering spirituality in occupational therapy practice. Canadian Journal of Occupational Therapy 61(2):95–101

Emmanuel E J, Emmanuel L L 1992 Four models of the physician–patient relationship. Journal of the American Medical Association 267(16):2221–2226

Fehrsen G S, Henbest R J 1993 In search of excellence. Expanding the patient-centred clinical method: a three stage assessment. Family Practice 10(1):49–54

Gage M 1994 The patient driven interdisciplinary care plan. Journal of Nursing Administration 24(4):26–35

Greenfield S, Kaplan S, Ware J E 1985 Expanding patient involvement in care. Annals of Internal Medicine 102:520–528

Grol R, de Maeseneer J, Whitfield M, Mokkink H 1990 Disease centred versus patient centred attitudes: comparison of general practitioners in Belgium, Britain and The Netherlands. Family Practice 7(2):100–103

Haig A J, Nagy A, LeBreck D B et al 1994 Patient oriented rehabilitation planning in a single visit: first year review of the quick program. Archives of Physical Medicine and Rehabilitation 75:172–176

Henbest R J, Fehrsen G S 1992 Patient-centredness: is it applicable outside the West? Its measurement and effect on outcomes. Family Practice 9(3):311–317

Henbest R J, Stewart M 1990 Patient-Centredness in the consultation 2: Does it really make a difference? Family Practice 7(1):28–33

Hobson S 1996 Being client centred when the client is cognitively impaired. Canadian Journal of Occupational Therapy 63(2):133–137

Law M, Baptiste S, Mills J 1995 Client centred practice: what does it mean and does it make a difference? Canadian Journal of Occupational Therapy 62(5):250–257

Levenstein J H, McCracken E C, McWhinney I R, Stewart M, Brown J B 1986 The patient centred clinical method 1. A model for the doctor patient interaction in family medicine. Family Practice 3(1):24–30

McColl M A, Pranger T 1994 Theory and practice in the guidelines for client centred practice. Canadian Journal of Occupational Therapy 61(5):250–259

McCracken E C, Stewart M A, Brown J B, McWhinney I R 1983 Patient centred care: the family practice model. Canadian Family Physician 29:2313–2316

Nuffield Institute 1995 Progress with patient focussed care in the United Kingdom. Nuffield Institute, University of Leeds

Reed K, Sanderson S R 1980 Concepts of occupational therapy. Williams and Wilkins, Baltimore

Richmond T S, Collican M, McKnew L B, Burton H 1994 Health care ethics forum '94: ethical care from the patient's perspective. American Association of Critical Care Nursing 5(3):308–312

Robinson N C 1991 A patient centred framework for restructuring care. Journal of Nursing Administration 21(9):29–34

Sherr Klein B 1997 Slow dance: a story of stroke, love and disability. Vintage Canada, Toronto

Speechley V 1992 Patients as partners. European Journal of Cancer Care 1(3):22–26

Stewart D, Harvey S 1990 Application of the guidelines for client centred practice to paediatrics. Canadian Journal of Occupational Therapy 57(2):88–94

Stewart M, Brown J B, Weston W W 1989 Patient centred interviewing. Part III. Five provocative questions. Canadian Family Physician 35:159–161

Stewart M, Belle Brown J, Weston W, McWhinney I, McWilliam C, Freeman T 1995 Patient centred medicine transforming the clinical method. Sage, London

Sumsion T 1993 Client centred practice: the true impact. Canadian Journal of Occupational Therapy 60(1):6–8

Sumsion T 1997 Environmental challenges and opportunities of client centred practice. British Journal of Occupational Therapy 60(2):53–56

Sumsion T 1999 A study to determine a British occupational therapy definition of client-centred practice. British Journal of Occupation Therapy 62: in press

Urbanowski R, Vargo J 1994 Spirituality, daily practice and the occupational performance model. Canadian Journal of Occupational Therapy 61(2):88–94

Western Alumni 1997 Learning to Care. University of Western Ontario, London

Weston W W, Brown J B, Stewart M A 1989 Patient centred interviewing. Part I: Understanding patients' experiences. Canadian Family Physician 35:147–151

Wilson J H, Hobbs H 1995 Therapeutic partnership: a model for clinical practice. Journal of Psychosocial Nursing 33(2):27–39

Wilson R A 1985 Client centred health education: a chance for provider change. Family and Community Health February: 1–4

World Health Organisation 1984 Discussion document on the concept and principles of health promotion. Canadian Public Health Association Health Digest 8:101–102

2

The client-centred approach

T. Sumsion

In order to implement client-centred practice, the process that leads to the achievement of goals must be understood. This chapter presents the views of four authors on the occupational therapy process. The traditional approach to intervention is discussed and contrasted with the client-centred process. This information provides the framework within which to consider detailed discussion in subsequent chapters.

Many pressures impact on the work of an occupational therapist. These pressures often absorb whatever time might otherwise be available for the planning and implementation of a creative approach for use with an individual or group of individuals. These same pressures also pose the threat that work with clients may become rote and systematic rather than individually tailored. It is therefore important that therapists consider the approach they use as well as the process that accompanies that approach and leads to a meaningful outcome for the client.

In this discussion the occupational therapy process refers to the specific stages in which a client and therapist engage from the moment the therapist is advised about the client to the time their work together ceases. These stages are enacted according to and guided by the therapist's chosen model or frame of reference. It is important to be consciously aware of all of the stages of the process to ensure that none is missed and all are used to the maximum benefit of the client.

VIEWS ON THE OCCUPATIONAL THERAPY PROCESS

The concept of a therapeutic process is not new to occupational therapists. In 1983 Reed and Sanderson outlined a problem-solving process model that followed seven stages. The first stage was the referral and initial evaluation, when the therapist gathered information about the client's occupational performance. Analysis then occurred to determine whether or not this person would benefit from occupational therapy intervention. The third stage was a formative evaluation to determine whether the person was receptive to the concept of occupational therapy. Next a plan was formulated that considered many aspects of intervention including goals, media and methods to be used. Then the programme was conducted, ensuring that the client understood what was taking place. The sixth step was a summative evaluation to determine whether changes should be made to the programme. Finally a decision was made to discharge the client and to arrange any other services that might be required (Reed and Sanderson 1983).

This problem-solving process model formed the basis for the work of the Canadian task force that designed the original Model of Occupational Performance. The client is actively involved in each of the seven stages of the occupational therapy process that accompanies the conceptual framework. The first stage is the referral when it is determined, through a review of the information received, whether or not the client would benefit from occupational therapy intervention. The criteria for making this decision will be determined by the programme within which the occupational therapist works. The second stage is assessment. Data are collected from a variety of sources both within and outside occupational therapy. Interviews, observations and specific standardised and non-standardised tools are components of the assessment which, for an occupational therapist, will focus on task functioning. A careful review of the accumulated information leads the therapist to a conclusion and recommendations for intervention which

are clearly documented. The assessment data are organised during the programme planning stage when all elements that would impact on the delivery of the programme are considered. Planning includes the choice of an appropriate model or frame of reference on which to base the intervention as well as the resources available to carry out the intervention. The plan is implemented in the intervention stage when the therapist and client work together to achieve the agreed goals. Occupational therapy goals relate to restoring, maintaining or developing function and preventing dysfunction. Re-evaluation of the client's progress occurs throughout the intervention in preparation for discharge, which is the fifth stage. At this point it is determined that the client will not gain anything further from the programme. Ideally the discharge plans have been part of the process from stage one rather than receiving attention only at this stage. It is also important to ensure that all aspects of the intervention are concluded, including the client–therapist relationship. Follow-up is the next stage but it is recognised that this is not always possible for an occupational therapist to do. The therapist's mandate may not include assessment of ongoing function or the ability to provide additional information that the client may require. The final stage is programme evaluation. The timing of this will vary according to the policies of the employer but it is important that some mechanism be in place to evaluate whether or not the intervention was effective. The employer in conjunction with the therapist should set criteria or standards to monitor the quality of each stage (Department of National Health and Welfare and Canadian Association of Occupational Therapists 1983).

Hagedorn (1995) refers to the occupational therapy process as case management. She reminds therapists that this process is not unique to occupational therapy and is based on concepts that are also adopted by other health professionals. Clinical reasoning and problem analysis are key components of this process. She outlines and discusses an additional six core processes of occupational therapy (Hagedorn 1995):

- Assessment and evaluation of individual potential
- Occupational analysis and adaptation
- Environmental analysis and adaptation
- Therapeutic use of self
- Implementation of therapy/intervention
- Resource management

These processes are fundamental to all interventions planned or carried out by an occupational therapist. They should be considered throughout all stages of the client-centred occupational therapy process, which is described as a linear undertaking but in reality is an ever-changing and fluid interactive chain of events.

The view of this process continues to evolve and be influenced by models of practice. Fearing et al (1997) have outlined an occupational performance process model as a guideline for therapists attempting to be client centred in their practice. The reader is referred to Chapter 10 for a pictorial outline of this process. This model supports client-centred practice and sees the therapist as an expert in both the process and the understanding of occupation. The first step is to name, validate and prioritise occupational performance problems and issues. In this beginning stage the therapist works with the client to identify issues of concern related to self-care, productivity and leisure. Problems are named and their order of importance is identified. The second step is the selection of potential intervention models. This stage supports the earlier comment that intervention is based on one or more theoretical approaches. The chosen approach will guide the methods used in both assessment and intervention. The third stage is the identification of occupational performance components and environmental conditions. A chosen assessment method is used to identify issues contributing to the client's occupational problems. In the fourth stage the therapist and client work together to identify skills and resources that the client can use to assist in the resolution of the acknowledged problems. Next, targeted outcomes are negotiated and action plans are developed. It is important that the therapist and client agree on the goals as little can be achieved by working

toward different outcomes. In the sixth stage the agreed plan is implemented through the use of meaningful occupations. Finally the occupational performance outcomes are evaluated. In keeping with the stages that accompanied the Model of Occupational Performance, these authors have recognised the importance of evaluating the effectiveness of the intervention. The Canadian Occupational Performance Measure (see Ch. 10) is an outcome measure based on a client-centred approach to evaluation.

TRADITIONAL APPROACH TO INTERVENTION

All occupational therapists adhere to a complete or modified process when working with clients, and most are familiar with the traditional approach. This process begins with the receipt of a referral as was outlined in the discussion of the process that accompanies the Model of Occupational Performance. This referral may either be specific to an individual client or a blanket referral that requires all clients in a particular programme to be seen by the occupational therapist. The information contained in this referral will also vary from being quite prescriptive, such as a directive to issue a particular piece of equipment, to fairly general, asking that the client be seen for an evaluation of functional problems. There will undoubtedly be a policy that accompanies the receipt of a referral indicating the amount of time within which the client must be seen.

The next step usually involves the therapist meeting with the client for an initial session. The contact usually begins with introductions and an explanation for the referral and the services that the therapist and the programme can offer. The discussion proceeds on to a more detailed review of the client's history and current problems. The therapist will also endeavour to gain an understanding of at least some of the environments in which the client is involved and which impact on occupational performance. The gathering of full information about relevant environments may necessitate a visit to the client's home. The therapist may proceed to conduct other specific assessments during this session or arrangements may be made for future meetings when this can occur.

Once the assessments are complete the therapist analyses the results and meets with the client again to outline what the programme can offer to assist with the resolution or improvement of the identified problems. The intervention is then carried out. Throughout the intervention the therapist is conducting ongoing evaluations to determine whether aspects of the intervention require modification because of changes in either the client or the circumstances. When either the goals of the intervention have been achieved or no further gains can be made, the intervention is terminated. It is unlikely within the health-care climate of today that a therapist will be permitted to contact the client again in a specified time to determine whether any further assistance is required. The reality is that, as soon as a client has been discharged from a programme, there is a waiting list of many more to take his or her place. If possible and appropriate the client will be referred to another programme to offer assistance in another environment, but the reality is that other programmes also will probably have a waiting list.

Evaluation is the final step to be considered. Most funding agencies now require that some form of individual or programme evaluation be undertaken. This may be in the form of audits, assessments of the client before and after therapy, or other forms of evaluative research. This final evaluation is enhanced by the evaluation that occurs throughout the process and influences revisions to the intervention. Overall this process is driven by a shortage of time and scarce resources which require the therapist to be as efficient as possible and to spend the minimum amount of time with each client.

CLIENT-CENTRED PROCESS

In contrast to the traditional approach, the client-centred process places the focus on the client rather than on the system that drives the intervention. The client-centred process is enabling. The therapist and client form a strong partnership to enable the attainment of the client's chosen goals. The client-centred process involves the following five stages:

- Referral
- Assessment and data gathering
- Client sets goals
- Partnership to attain goals
- Evaluation

Referral

The stages of a client-centred process may also begin with the receipt of a referral that the therapist reviews with the client to determine the suggested direction of the intervention. The client's views on and understanding of the reason for the referral are sought in the initial meeting. The referral does not direct the intervention; rather it provides the reason for the initial meeting with the client and the impetus for the process to begin. Negotiation with the referral source may be necessary if the client's views of his or her involvement in the process differ from those presented in the referral.

Assessment and data gathering

The initial meeting with the client is used to gather assessment information and to explain the parameters of the programme to which the client has been referred. Issues such as number or length of sessions and programme mandates should be identified early in the process. The client-centred approach should also be discussed at this time. This approach warrants some initial discussion as it will be new and unique for most clients. The effectiveness of the entire process will be enhanced at this early stage if the client understands the key issues of this working relationship that will evolve into a partnership. The focus of the initial meeting is on the client rather than on the limitations for this particular programme or the system at large. The therapist discusses the client's views of the problem for which the referral was made and goals and wishes concerning change. It must be recognised that these goals and wishes may not be in total agreement with either the reason for referral or the therapist's choice of the emphasis for the intervention. Methods of gathering the necessary information, either about the presenting problems or about possible resources to assist with the problem, are agreed and a subsequent meeting time is arranged.

Tools are emerging to assist with the client-centred focus of this initial meeting and assessment. The Canadian Occupational Performance Measure (COPM) is discussed in Chapter 10 and serves as both an initial interview guide and an outcome measure. The Client Centred Occupational Performance Initial Interview (CCOPII) was designed for use with clients who have mental health problems and are living in the community. It is a semistructured interview based on occupational performance (Orford 1995). Clients are asked about things that are troubling them and problems that prevent them from doing what they want to do, with particular emphasis on self-care, rest or relaxation, work, leisure and relationships. The interview is framed in both present and historical contexts, and focuses on strengths as well as problems. Short-term goals to address the issues the client identifies are agreed and a time for a review of progress toward these goals is determined. These are two examples of client-centred tools, but therapists may be able to use other assessments in a client-centred way.

Client sets goals

In the next stage the therapist and client meet again to discuss all the information that has been gathered. Time must be spent to ensure that the client understands the information and has ample opportunity both to ask questions and to have them answered. A further challenge for the therapist is to ensure that the client has all of the information that is necessary to make a decision about the goals and methods of intervention. This may require the presentation of information in a variety of formats and over a series of sessions. Information may originally be presented verbally and then in writing, or perhaps by means of a demonstration either in person or on video. The client needs the opportunity to take information home for further consideration and to assist with the formulation of questions for future sessions. Types of information will relate to client strengths and problems, available financial and service resources, consideration of the environment and other people involved, and the therapist's expertise. At this point the parameters of the programme that were discussed in the initial session may have to be reviewed. The client needs to understand the realities and limitations of the available resources before determining the goals for intervention. The client-centred approach requires that time and energy be dedicated to the analysis and understanding of the assessment information before the goals are set. The client then sets the goals. This is potentially the most important step in this process. The client owns the goals as she or he is the one who will benefit directly when they are met. The therapist will not benefit directly so does not have the right to establish a plan without the client's direct participation (Nicholson & Tobaben-Wyssmann 1984). The goals need to be stated clearly in a format that allows their achievement to be reviewed. Again, time must be dedicated to the discussion of these goals to ensure that they are clearly understood by everyone who is involved in or impacted by them.

Partnership to attain goals

The therapist and client now work in partnership to achieve the goals. The therapist has considerable knowledge to contribute to this process but must also become an educator and facilitator to remove obstacles to the attainment of the agreed goals. Updated information must be provided on an ongoing basis but particularly when there are new decisions to be made (Sumsion 1993). Ongoing evaluation also occurs throughout the process, and therapist and client agree when the point is reached to re-evaluate the goals and then to terminate the intervention. As was discussed previously, therapists must be as mindful of terminating their relationship with the client as they are of terminating other aspects of the therapeutic relationship.

Evaluation

Forms of evaluation are the same as those for the traditional approach. Hopefully the one difference will be that the client's views will be included in an official way rather than relying on the criteria for success established by the professionals. In Chapter 9 Marie Gage suggests some methods of evaluation when working with clients with physical disabilities. The COPM (presented in more detail in Chapter 10) which was referred to in the assessment stage is revisited here and clients rescore their goals according to their satisfaction and performance. There are also many other methods of evaluation that could be used including a review of the established goals, audits of both the process and specific interventions, and use of a range of other outcome measures that are being developed to meet the demands of this stage of the process.

CONCLUSION

All the stages of this process raise many issues that relate to the realities faced by both the therapist and client, and that will be discussed in subsequent chapters. There are some similarities between a traditional and a client-centred approach. However, the major difference relates to the role of the client throughout the process and his or her place as a key player in all stages. The partnership that is a key ingredient of the client-centred process cannot occur unless this involvement becomes a major focus of the intervention. The occupational therapy process should not be treated superficially. Rather, there should always be clear evidence that this is a carefully considered process with clear documentation of the contributions and responsibilities of all members of the partnership at each stage of the process.

REFERENCES

Department of National Health and Welfare and Canadian Association of Occupational Therapists 1983 Guidelines for the client centred practice of occupational therapy. Department of National Health and Welfare, Ottawa

Fearing V G, Law M, Clark J 1997 An occupational performance process model: fostering client and therapist alliances. Canadian Journal of Occupational Therapy 64(1):7–15

Hagedorn R 1995 Occupational therapy perspectives and processes. Churchill Livingstone, Edinburgh

Nicholson J R, Tobaben-Wyssmann S 1984 Client centred rehabilitation: a method for setting realistic goals to meet client needs. Journal of Rehabilitation November/December:39–41,72

Orford J 1995 Community mental health: the development of the CCOPII, a client centred occupational performance initial interview. British Journal of Occupational Therapy 58(5):190–196

Reed K L, Sanderson S R 1983 Concepts of occupational therapy. Williams and Wilkins, Baltimore

Sumsion T 1993 Client centred practice: the true impact. Canadian Journal of Occupational Therapy 60(1):6–8

3

Environmental considerations

T. Sumsion

This chapter presents a general introduction to current thinking about a range of environments within occupational therapy, and the approach taken by several prominent authors is presented. A case study provides a focus for the discussion about the cultural, economic, legal, physical, political and social environments. These environments are interconnected but are discussed separately to facilitate consideration of their individual importance.

The environment is receiving increasing attention within occupational therapy literature. This emergence is an important recognition of the increasing number of challenges faced by clients from a variety of environments. One example is seen in the revised International Classification of Impairment, Disability and Handicap. This circular model replaces disability with activity and recognises the importance of context for the client when engaging in activity within the environment (Chard 1997). The therapist's role is to work with environmental issues to facilitate the achievement of the client's goals or to remove the barriers that inhibit attainment of these goals. The purpose of this chapter is not to reveal all that must be known about these complex environments. Rather, a focus on a case study will help therapists consider issues that must be addressed in relation to a variety of environments when engaging with any client.

There are many complex and interconnected concepts related to the environment that afford opportunities for performance (Kielhofner 1995). Humans seek congenial environments that are a good match for them, and will change the environment to reach this state. Humans are free to choose how they act in the environment, which will influence their freedom to make meaningful choices (Capitman & Sciegaj 1995). The environment also presses for occupational behaviour by placing demands on the individual. This press may be exerted by the way the environment is arranged, the expectations of others in the environment and the systems created to deal with specific procedures. This press can either support or work against an individual's participation (Law 1991). The amount of impact any environment has will depend on several aspects of the person, including values, roles and habits. Therefore therapists should be aware that the environment influences occupational performance. Occupational therapy involves environmentally based strategies that impact on the occupational performance of clients in everyday life. 'Therapists cannot understand occupational performance unless they also understand the environment in which it occurs' (Kielhofner 1995). This is such an important concept that we 'owe our very humanness and our most essential selves to our environments' (Kielhofner 1995). In the Model of Human Occupation it is clear that environments influence behaviour and impact on occupational choice.

Occupational therapists are skilled at adapting the environment. First therapists need to analyse the environment and its impact on the individual to identify the causes of maladaptation. Then the environment can be adapted to promote access and facilitate performance. The level of stimulation provided by the environment must also be considered (Hagedorn 1997).

Law (1991) has written extensively about issues related to the environment. She defines the environment as 'those contexts and situations which occur outside individuals and elicit responses from them'. A person–environment–occupation clinical model of occupational performance builds on concepts presented in the Model of Occupational Performance (Law et al 1996). The three components of this clinical model are the individual's skills, environmental supports and barriers, and occupational demands. Occupational performance

occurs when the three elements overlap. The components interact continually, and individual components are often in a constant state of change. This model defines the environment broadly so that all aspects can be considered. It also recognises that the environment is not static and is often more amenable to change than the person. The contribution of the occupational therapist is to maximise the fit between what the client wants to do, needs to do and is capable of doing. This cannot be accomplished unless the elements within the person are integrated with the environmental context (Baum & Law 1997).

SPECIFIC ENVIRONMENTS

The separation between environments is artificial as all are interconnected and different aspects of each will influence the others at different times. There is also interdependence between the person and the environment, so any attempt at separation is artificial (Law et al 1996). The focus on individual environments will also shift to meet the needs of the client (Sumsion 1997).

This interdependence between the environments is recognised. However, this discussion will present six separate environments to facilitate the appreciation of the importance of each one. The challenge presented by client-centred practice is to consider all environments in relation to the issues relevant to the individual. Therapists are failing in their obligation to clients if the influence of each environment is not considered in the initial stages of the interaction. Some environments will be quickly dismissed and others will become the focus of the intervention.

The six environments to be discussed are those presented by the Model of Occupational Performance (Canadian Association of Occupational Therapists 1991, 1993). These are the cultural, economic, legal, physical, political and social environments. They are presented here in alphabetical order simply to facilitate their location rather than to imply any hierarchy. Each environment will be discussed in the context of the case of Mr C.

The case of Mr C

Mr and Mrs C are both 83 years old and have been married for 56 years. They have no children and live in a two-storey, 100-year-old house on her family's farm. The bathroom is on the upper level. Most of the land is rented but there is still a large yard and garden for them to maintain. Mrs C has run an antique business for many years and still does so on a part-time basis. Mr C is an accountant. Both Mr and Mrs C are licensed drivers. Mr C began to experience extreme low back pain. After extensive tests and the involvement of several doctors he underwent surgery to fuse two discs in his lower back and emergency surgery two days later to relieve spinal pressure. Mr C was in intensive care for two weeks, spent some time on a surgical ward and was subsequently transferred to a spinal cord rehabilitation facility. Their home is 100 miles from the rehabilitation centre so Mrs C could visit only when someone was able to drive her or she was able to take the train on her own. On admission to the rehabilitation facility Mr C was unable to walk, turn himself over in bed, eat or dress independently, and could not write or use the telephone. He worked extremely hard at his rehabilitation and three months later could walk with a walker, feed himself, dress his upper body and use the telephone.

Four months after his admission to the rehabilitation centre Mr C was able to return home for a five-day visit. The staff at the centre made arrangements with the local home care office for an occupational therapist to visit the home to discuss environmental barriers, a nurse to visit daily and a homemaker to come twice for three hours while Mr C was there. The home care coordinator at the rehabilitation facility assumed these arrangements would work simply because the request had been made. In reality the local home care coordinator was not cooperative, Mrs C had trouble getting the hospital bed she had ordered, the occupational therapist refused to understand the significance to this couple of the age of their home and their unwillingness to renovate, and the community nurse arrived late at night. However, in spite of these obstacles Mr C's visit home was a success, as were several subsequent visits. He was discharged from the centre a few months later and continued to make steady progress. A couple of years later he is driving the car, walking up the stairs to the bathroom and has basically resumed his independent life. The rehabilitation team, his friends and family are all amazed at the determination and strength of will of both Mr and Mrs C that enabled them to overcome this major life challenge and resume their busy life.

CULTURAL ENVIRONMENT

Culture is an abstract concept. It involves learned and shared patterns of perceiving and adapting to the world (Fitzgerald et al 1997). Culture includes beliefs, values, norms, customs and behaviours that are shared by a group or a society (Kielhofner 1995). Therapists must not allow their own cultural background or personal values and biases to determine their approach to a client. Culture can influence a client's symptoms as it has an impact on emotions. This needs to be considered when working with clients in a mental health setting as cultural expectations and socialisation impact on a person's emotional response. Distress is interpreted within a social order that is established by a culture (Kirmayer 1989).

A first review of this case might not reveal any cultural issues. Mr and Mrs C live in the country of their birth in a location where they have been for many years. But there are issues that must be addressed. Everyone is part of a variety of cultures and subcultures (Sumsion 1997). In this case the rural subculture must be considered as people in this culture simply get on with dealing with the challenges presented by life. The elements are a constant challenge with which rural people deal. In order to survive, they have to be independent but at the same time they are also willing to help a neighbour. In this culture you only have to ask for help once and it is provided. The men on neighbouring farms readily provided assistance with problems of wheelchair access and troublesome catheters. Others drove several miles to the pharmacy to collect prescriptions and checked to see whether other provisions were required.

The sick role is also an important consideration when discussing the cultural environment. Clearly this couple was not prepared to adopt this role. Independence and function are important to them and they were determined to maintain this state. The importance of family within any culture must also be considered. This couple does not have any children nor any family close enough or well enough to be of assistance.

A major cultural issue relates to the occupational therapist and her lack of understanding of the importance of culture to this couple. She did not acknowledge that they live in a heritage home which they were not prepared to alter. Nor did she acknowledge the strength of character of an elderly rural couple who are very assertive. They have good ideas and know what is best for them. They do not respond well to being told what to do. Overall this therapist did not use a client-centred approach.

ECONOMIC ENVIRONMENT

No literature was found that discusses the economic environment in relation to clients. However, there are daily reminders in the press about the financial constraints faced by services and programmes with which clients engage. These financial limitations will impact on clients, who may not have access to the services they choose. Funding for long-term care facilities is of particular concern as private owners attempt to minimise expenditures and state-funded services face budgets that do not meet the costs of operating the programme. Mr and Mrs C have an established business so there were no immediate financial concerns. However, they will not be able to keep the business going forever, so must be aware of financial issues in order to support their lifestyle as long as necessary. They have paid taxes for many years and have the right to access the same services as others that are less financially independent. The inability of the home care coordinator at the rehabilitation centre to visit the home and ascertain that the requested services were being provided may have been due to limited budgets for travel.

LEGAL ENVIRONMENT

The legal environment is gaining prominence as clients are increasingly involved in legal matters such as accident or insurance claims and malpractice suits. Clients are also becoming more educated about the legal environment and their rights to access funds to support their needs. It is impossible for therapists to maintain current knowledge about all legal matters, but they must have access to legal advice (Sumsion 1997). Therapists also need to be aware of their own rights and the laws that govern their

programmes in order to protect themselves against legal action.

Mr and Mrs C might have benefited from advice about the services to which they were entitled and what action to take when these services were not readily available or were not offered in a suitable manner. All clients need to know their rights but this is becoming an increasingly important issue in relation to the elderly. Following Mr C's serious illness the couple was aware of the need to ensure that their legal affairs were in order and went to see a lawyer to update their wills and to put systems in place to ensure that their wishes were respected. Their assertiveness and business skill allowed them to deal with their legal concerns effectively but other clients may not be as fortunate.

PHYSICAL ENVIRONMENT

The physical environment is the traditional domain of occupational therapists and the one with which they are most familiar. The emphasis on barrier-free design often focuses attention on this environment. The physical environment can be divided into natural components, such as the countryside, and built components, such as buildings. Natural objects such as trees and fabricated objects such as clothes and cars are also part of the physical environment (Kielhofner 1995). Law (1991) supports this description by discussing the components of a built environment including buildings, playgrounds, streets and pavements. Creation of the physical environment is often influenced by societal values. 'Society has created an environment which severely constrains the daily activities and participation of many people' (Law 1991). Many barriers in the physical environment inhibit independence. Therefore it is important that occupational therapists are able to assess this environment accurately. Iwarsson and Isacsson (1996) recognised the importance of reliable assessments to unify the person, disability and function, and created the Enabler to address this concern. It measures individual functional limitation, dependence on mobility devices and environmental barriers.

There are many physical issues to be discussed in relation to Mr and Mrs C. The most obvious one is the lack of sensitivity of the occupational therapist whose only approach to their needs was to recommend renovation of their environment. She failed to recognise the cultural implications of this suggestion and to work with the couple to devise solutions that were suitable to them. She did not recommend a commode chair or simple rearrangements to the ground floor to create a bedroom for Mr C. Mrs C was left to find the resources to create the necessary environmental changes. Safety is of course an important issue to consider. The therapist may have been focused on this when she recommended a renovation to address the safety of Mr C going up stairs. However, she failed to listen to him when he said he would be able to go up the stairs soon. She also failed to facilitate ways that he could reach this goal. His determination allowed him to reach the goal in spite of the health professionals rather than with their assistance. The therapist also failed to assist him with the fabricated objects in his environment and did not address issues such as how to shave or wash independently. The physical environment may be the focus of occupational therapy but there is no excuse for ignoring the client's wishes and goals in the process. Occupational therapy is a creative profession that, in partnership with the client, can create exciting solutions to physical challenges.

POLITICAL ENVIRONMENT

Individual practitioners do not have a strong tradition of political involvement. However, politics are real and impact on the daily lives of clients. The decisions of local councils about the allocation of funding for accessible public transport or ramped pathways impact on clients. The other members of the partnership, people with disabilities, have traditionally had little political power but this is changing rapidly. Of particular relevance here is the growing political awareness and power of the elderly. Therapists need to be aware of political issues and how they impact on clients and to support client-led initiatives that endeavour to make all environments more accessible to

clients (Sumsion 1997). Therapists may need to enhance their roles as advocates and facilitators to ensure that positive changes occur. Mrs C is particularly assertive, so no political intervention was required, but that does not excuse the failure to evaluate this aspect of the environment to ascertain what issues should be addressed.

SOCIAL ENVIRONMENT

The social environment is complex and has many different components. This environment is composed of social groups, such as family and co-workers, and occupational forms, such as dressing or fishing (Kielhofner 1995). Mr and Mrs C do not have a large family but they do have many friends who are part of their chosen family. Many volunteers, such as the driver from the Red Cross who drove Mrs C to the city to visit her husband, also became friends and formed an important part of this environment. Their farm is on the edge of a small village where many people have lived all their lives. This longevity forms close social ties that are strengthened in times when assistance is needed. Their antique business has a national reputation which also enlarges their social circle and assists the village by giving it a position of prominence.

Social roles must also be considered. Hospitals are a social environment where those who are ill are expected to conform. In the hospital environment Mr C was not expected to make a full recovery. However, at home he was viewed as a vital man who had a role as a husband and farm manager. In this environment there was faith in his strength and abilities and he responded to this in very positive ways. A positive social environment accepts the person for what they are and encourages them to be whatever they wish. Today Mr C enjoys his garden, which he plans and organises although a friend does the heavy work. He drives his car and enjoys a rich life where all his roles are supported and encouraged.

CONCLUSION

This case discussion has emphasised the need for therapists to become familiar with assessments that will enable them to evaluate the influence of all environments. Each of the six environments must be considered in light of the individual circumstances presented by each client. Some environments will emerge as being of greater significance than other environments, but all must be considered. These environments have been discussed in isolation to stress their importance but in reality there is considerable overlap between them. For example, the friends from the rural environment who were so willing to be of assistance form part of both the cultural and social environments. Therapists also work within a changing environment that presents increasing amounts of press that will influence their ability to support the client's goals in each environment. However, this does not lessen their responsibility to consider all environments and to work with the client to establish a list of priority issues that will influence goal attainment.

REFERENCES

Baum C M, Law M 1997 Occupational therapy practice: focusing on occupational performance. American Journal of Occupational Therapy 51(4):277–288

Canadian Association of Occupational Therapists 1991 Occupational therapy guidelines for client centred practice. CAOT Publications ACE, Toronto

Canadian Association of Occupational Therapists 1993 Occupational therapy guidelines for client centred practice. CAOT Publications ACE, Toronto

Capitman J, Sciegaj M 1995 A contextual approach for understanding individual autonomy in managed community long term care. Gerontologist 35(4):533–540

Chard G 1997 Impairment, activity and participation. British Journal of Occupational Therapy 60(9):383

Fitzgerald M H, Mullavey-O'Byrne C, Clemson L 1997 Cultural issues from practice. Australian Occupational Therapy Journal 44:1–21

Hagedorn R 1997 Foundations for practice in occupational therapy. Churchill Livingstone, Edinburgh

Iwarsson S, Isacsson A 1996 Development of a novel instrument for occupational therapy assessment of the physical environment in the home – a methodologic study on 'The Enabler'. Occupational Therapy Journal of Research 16(4):227–244

Kielhofner G 1995 A model of human occupation; theory and application. Williams and Wilkins, Baltimore

Kirmayer L 1989 Cultural variations in the response to psychiatric disorders and emotional distress. Social Science Medicine 29(3):327–339

Law M 1991 The environment: a focus for occupational therapy. Canadian Journal of Occupational Therapy 58(4):171–180

Law M, Cooper B, Strong S, Stewart D, Rigby P, Letts L 1996 The person–environment–occupation model: a transactive approach to occupational performance. Canadian Journal of Occupational Therapy 63(1):9–23

Sumsion T 1997 Environmental challenges and opportunities of client-centred practice. British Journal of Occupational Therapy 60(2):53–56

4

Implementation issues

T. Sumsion

This chapter discusses the issues that add challenge to the implementation of client-centred practice. These issues include the importance of clarifying who is the client, the shift of power from the therapist to the client, the therapist as an educator, client choice and safety, and client-centred language. The barriers to client-centred practice presented by the therapist, the client and the working environment are also discussed.

There are many issues a therapist must address before implementing a client-centred approach effectively. Many therapists believe that client-centred practice is inherent in occupational therapy, which has a tradition of using a holistic approach. 'From its inception occupational therapy has viewed the human being as a complex mix of internal physical, psychological, social and cultural variables living within an equally dynamic environmental mixture of social, cultural, interpersonal, economic and political variables' (Kielhofner 1985). Therefore it may appear that no alterations are required as, by its very nature, occupational therapy is client centred. It is true that if all aspects of the Model of Occupational Performance are addressed with every client then a truly holistic approach has been used. However, there are many issues related to both the application of the individual components of the model and the overall philosophy of client-centred practice that must be considered if one is to be a client-centred therapist.

DEFINITION OF CLIENT

The first issue to be considered is the definition of the term client. The discussion of whether the people with whom occupational therapists work should be called patients or clients has been ongoing for a number of years. In 1984 Reilly cautioned therapists that changing the terminology from patient to client was very serious. She was concerned that this switch in terminology would in fact threaten the survival of the profession. Other authors entered this debate and defined a patient as a recipient of services who, as an individual, was waiting for or under medical care and treatment. In contrast a client was a consumer of services, a patron or customer, or a person under the protection of another. These authors were concerned that therapists who used the term client were moving from a relationship based on a moral and ethical tradition to one based on a legal and economic foundation (Sharrott and Yerxa 1985). They were also concerned that occupational therapists were in danger of losing the profession's identification with service and caring if they climbed on the corporate bandwagon. Herzberg responded to this argument a few years later by pointing out that Sharrott and Yerxa had neglected to mention that there are other definitions of both patient and client. A patient can also be defined as one who is acted upon and a client as a person who engages the professional services of another. A client has the right to demand information and is free to voice an opinion, and a patient is told what to do and actively seeks help (Herzberg 1990).

The Canadian Association of Occupational Therapists (CAOT) originally defined a client as 'a recipient of occupational therapy services' (CAOT 1991). As the concepts related to client-centred practice developed, it became clear that it was important to determine who was the client before an intervention began. In fact the client may not be the identified patient, so it is important to consider broadening the definition of client to incorporate others, including family members, significant others, community agencies, or carers and partners (Gustafson 1991). This expansion is an important issue when working with children or clients with cognitive impairment. This expanded thinking is clearly articulated in a recent document from CAOT (1997) which defines client as:

Individuals with occupational problems arising from medical conditions, transitional difficulties, or environmental barriers or clients may be organisations that influence the occupational performance of particular groups or populations.

There is no ready definition of client that will apply to every situation in which occupational therapists work. It is important for therapists to realise that the client may not at all times be the same person or the person who was referred to them. Expanded thinking is required to move beyond the usual determination of who is the client to include significant others in the client's environment. Therapists who are committed to applying a client-centred approach must avoid the decision that this approach cannot be used simply because obstacles are presented by the definition of the client. These obstacles might include issues faced by the identified client including an inability to communicate, to make decisions or readily to understand the information the therapist is providing. These situations require a broader definition of the client so that all the exciting aspects of client-centred practice can be activated.

Inherent in applying a client-centred approach is the acceptance of the term 'client'. The client is the person who chooses to be involved in the process as he or she is the one in need of the therapist's expertise. A therapist engages lawyers, builders or accountants to solve problems related to their areas of expertise and a client comes to a therapist for the same reasons. Everyone expects the people they engage to treat them with respect, to use their expertise to outline the available options and then to facilitate the necessary actions to implement the chosen options. In client-centred practice the element of choice may be less relevant as the client rarely faces a health or disability issue by choice. However, this does not lessen the reality that they are engaging with an expert who can advise them on the available options for reaching the desired goal. If a therapist cannot accept a person's right to be a client and all that this right entails then he or she cannot be a client-centred therapist.

POWER

Another issue to be considered before implementing a client-centred approach is the question of power. All professional relationships contain an element of power, and those wishing to implement a client-centred approach must consider the balance of power. Occupational therapists do not traditionally view themselves as people with power. If the reverse were true there would not continue to be discussions about either role erosion or the need to define clearly the place of the occupational therapist in various employment settings. However, occupational therapy is a health-care profession that, in the eyes of the consumer, holds considerable power.

Power over

It is important that the concept of power be clearly understood before considering the influence of power in interactions with clients. The traditional dictionary definition describes power as the possession of control, authority or influence over others. Henderson (1994), in a discussion of the power of knowledge, describes day-to-day power which places one person in a position of power over another. The concept of power over another person also influences behaviour and decisions of others to obey or conform and 'encompasses control, competitiveness, authority and leadership' (Raatikainen 1994). Power over is attributed to a sense of strength and creativity rather than weakness and inferiority (Hokanson Hawks 1991). Each of these authors places the emphasis on strength, control and competitiveness, which supports the idea that health professionals do have power over clients and that power certainly influences goal attainment. Gerhardt (1989) takes this discussion one step further by describing medicine as 'a self propelled power conscious body'. Hopefully this phrase does not also describe occupational therapy.

Language is also the medium of power. A medical vocabulary can be very confusing to clients and hence places the therapist in a position of power over the client (Gerhardt 1989). Simple language should be used in the provision of information to clients and time should be taken to ensure that all components of any discussion or written material have been understood.

Therapists may operationalise their power over people in a variety of ways. Expertise and power can be used to suppress and control the client's wishes to fit with the referral request; to control available funding for equipment; to refuse access to information the therapist decides would be harmful; to deny family participation in treatment; to limit available choices; and to deny someone the right to return home when the therapist determines that they cannot function independently. This power may be at its strongest in psychiatry where professionals hold people in a setting against their will. Therapists do have power over clients and may use their ability and knowledge to get the client to do something he or she would not otherwise have done (Hokanson Hawks 1991). Therefore power cannot be ignored and warrants careful consideration in any intervention but particularly in those that are meant to be client centred.

Power to

Rather than exerting power over clients therapists should be attempting to give power to them, particularly in a client-centred interaction. Giving power to people relates to effectiveness and the ability to set goals, achieve objectives and effect outcomes (Raatikainen 1994). Power is about giving control to individuals (Swaffield 1990).

Law et al (1995) outline the core concepts by defining power as a process by which the client and therapist achieve together what neither could achieve alone. Communication and participation in decision-making is the way to share power (Rogers 1983).

In summary, the defining attributes of power are (Hokanson Hawks 1991):

- the actual or potential ability or capacity to achieve objectives or attain goals
- an interpersonal process
- mutual establishment of goals and the means to achieve the goals
- mutually working toward goals.

All these points support the basic concepts inherent in client-centred practice. The client-centred process is no longer therapist led and therefore the power is no longer assigned to the therapist. Rather it is the client who directs the process and therefore has the power. Once this power is understood and accepted, clients become equal partners in health care and can foster their own health rather then always seeking professional help. The challenge for the professional is to accept the client's interpretation of the problem and theories related to it, and to take these interpretations seriously.

Implementation challenges

A client-centred approach requires therapists to surrender power but there is a certain threat attached to training others to do what a therapist was trained to do. If therapists train families or clients to treat themselves, then will the servant become the master? The traditional approach places the therapist as the helper in the stronger position over the person being helped. However, if the relationship is turned into a true partnership then the power that is gained by combining skills and wishes is a force with which others must reckon.

Another issue often raised by therapists relates to a lack of clarity about their role if they relinquish power and let the client have the control. The danger they see is that the therapist may not be needed. This is not the case because of the importance of facilitating the acceptance of responsibility through education. Client education becomes a critical role for therapists attempting to be client centred and as such assisting the client with the process of assuming power. Education is an important concept in any therapeutic relationship but within a client-centred approach education must be ongoing.

One of the core skills in assuming power is decision-making. Decisions cannot be made unless all the necessary information is available and understood.

Consideration must also be given to the possibility that the client does not want this power. This may be true, but it is not a decision a therapist should make in the initial stage of working with the client. However, this may be the conclusion the therapist and client reach as the intervention proceeds. The aim for the therapist is to use power effectively within a client-centred approach by asking questions so the client is a partner and not fearful of giving the wrong answer. The therapist should also really listen to clients and help them tune into the therapist's knowledge, and check back to ensure the client understands the information given to them and that the suggestions will work for them (Swaffield 1990).

Power skills can be obtained only through a working relationship that includes trust, knowledge, communication, concern, caring respect, courtesy and self-confidence. All relationships with clients are complex and power is a reality that adds to the complexity. If therapists truly wish to be client centred then they have to surrender power or they are only giving lip service to being client centred.

This means that therapists may:

- have to tailor programmes so that the issues being addressed are those that are important to the client rather than to the therapist
- have to help clients end their days in their own homes
- have to advocate for clients who are labelled as difficult because they will not comply with treatment that is not directed toward their goals
- need to be supporters of the self-help movement which meets the needs of clients that therapists are unable to address
- have to express views that differ from those of the other members of the multidisciplinary team.

Clients will set goals that seem unreasonable but they need to be helped to work toward those goals. An 80-year-old man needs help to drive again rather than the creation of obstructions simply because this goal appears unreasonable. A disabled mother needs creative solutions that will allow her to bottle-feed her child rather than being told to accept that others will do this for her. A troubled adolescent needs help to find alternative educational organisations rather than being told he must conform to the system. These may be radical examples, but the challenge of client-centred practice is to facilitate by the transfer of power rather than to obstruct by maintaining power.

The overriding skill that will make all this happen is communication – true, in-depth, open and honest communication. Only this will allow the therapist to understand what clients really want and need, and enable them to understand the realities of the system that may either facilitate or impede attainment of the desired goal.

THERAPIST AS EDUCATOR

It has previously been established that clients cannot make the necessary decisions unless they have all the relevant information. Ideally clients should always be given sufficient information to enable them to make informed decisions (College of Occupational Therapists 1995). The challenge for the therapist is to present this information in a way that is clearly understood by the client. This necessitates skilful communication abilities to assess which method of education will be most successful with various clients. Some will respond more effectively to written information while others will need the information described or demonstrated. Some will want to take the information home to discuss with others before making a decision. Clients are also becoming generally more informed as a result of access to the Internet and will be entering the process as more informed consumers (Richards 1998). In this situation therapists must be prepared to work with information that is presented to them and which may challenge their knowledge base or beliefs and values.

There is a connection between patient satisfaction and compliance in medicine and there is no reason to believe these same issues do not apply to other disciplines. Epstein et al (1993) discuss patient education as part of their model for a medical interview that will enhance satisfaction. When educating patients about illness it is important to elicit their ideas, check their baseline information and understanding, and elicit questions from them. Education is also important during the negotiation which determines the focus of the intervention. Again it is important to check understanding and to elicit the patient's preferences and commitments. Motivation will be enhanced if solutions are negotiated. Timing is also a crucial factor in the transmission of information. The client under considerable stress may not be able to absorb the knowledge required before making a decision (Deber 1994). Therapists must be sensitive to this stress and ensure that the provision of information acknowledges and accommodates the realities of the information being received. Communication is a crucial factor in education. If therapists listen and respond at the appropriate level then learning is enhanced for both the therapist and the client.

CLIENT CHOICE

Client choice was identified as an important consideration in the assumption of power but it remains important throughout all stages of the client-centred process. Clients may ultimately decide that they do not want to make the necessary decisions but would rather have the clinician set the goals and design the intervention for reaching those goals. However, a therapist who is truly client centred begins the process by providing all opportunities for the client to be the decision-maker, and it is only after careful discussion and negotiation that responsibility is removed from the client. Even the decision to not be the decision-maker cannot be made until all the necessary information has been provided. A therapist who decides to change the company from which car insurance is purchased cannot choose an alternative company until considerable research has been done and a variety of quotes received. Likewise clients cannot make decisions until they have all the necessary information that informs the available choices.

Clients are the experts about their own strengths and problems. Only they can truly understand what it is like to live their lives. Therefore they have a right to receive the information they need to make choices about how to confront these problems (Law et al 1995). Clients' views of the goals they want to achieve may also change over time. These changes require new information so that new decisions can be made. Final decisions about goals and the amount of energy to be expended to reach them can be determined only by the person directly involved (Mold et al 1991). Richards (1998) quotes the director of the King's Fund, who says that people want unbiased, current information about their illness and the risks and benefits of various interventions. This indicates that people are ready to make important and difficult choices.

CLIENT-CENTRED LANGUAGE

The application of client-centred practice requires the adoption of new language. Few new words are required but the pattern of word usage must be changed. Consider the words a therapist following the traditional approach to intervention would use when meeting with a client for the first time. It is likely that conversation would include a phrase such as: 'You are here because the consultant asked me to see you'. In client-centred practice this phrase would not be used. Rather the client would be asked why she was there so that her role as decision-maker might be established immediately. In a subsequent meeting to discuss the results of the assessment the therapist might traditionally have said: 'based on the results of the assessment here are the goals that we will be working toward'. In the client-centred approach the results would be discussed with the client rather than presented to him. Following receipt of all the necessary information, provided in a way the client can understand, the client then determines the goals for the intervention. Words must support actions. The actions necessary to be truly client-centred will not occur if the process does not begin with and continue to include the words that convey a commitment to this approach and the client's central role throughout the process.

BARRIERS TO CLIENT-CENTRED PRACTICE

Obstacles to the implementation of client-centred practice may be presented by the therapist, the client or the working environment (Law et al 1995). There are many barriers in each of these categories and their strength and relationship to one another will depend on the situation in which they occur. This discussion will identify several barriers but focus on those that are of greatest and most common concern.

Therapist barriers

Client safety

Therapists have a responsibility to ensure that goals set for intervention are safe and that no harm will come to the client. (Additional thoughts on this topic are presented by Marie Gage in Chapter 9.) This is relatively easy to achieve in the traditional approach to intervention as the therapist uses professional judgement to determine what is safe. However, the potential definitely exists in a client-centred approach for the client to determine goals that the therapist thinks are unsafe or that entail unnecessary risk (Law et al 1995). There is no easy answer to this dilemma. If clients have the right to make decisions about their plans, and if the therapist has provided all of the necessary information to ensure that clients understand the risks of their decision, then clients have the right to make a seemingly unsafe choice (Clemens et al 1994).

It is also possible that the therapist will be reluctant to take risks to support the client's goals (Hobson 1996). An increasing amount of press coverage is being given to clients who want to choose to die and to have someone assist them to do so. This choice is at the pinnacle of decision-making and each person must grapple with his or her own values and beliefs in relation to this decision. Hopefully occupational therapists will not have to enter the debate at this level but they will have to make decisions that could impact on a person's life. For example, an elderly client's choice to return home to live independently may clash with the occupational therapist's concerns about the safety of this decision. There may be concerns related to falls down stairs, burns when lighting gas appliances, or medication management. Unfortunately therapists do have to be concerned about issues of liability, particularly those related to decisions that could be interpreted as supporting an unsafe decision. However, if they document clearly the information that was given to the client, the discussion of the analysis of that information, the fact that the client indicated the information was understood and the implications of the decision the client has made, then perhaps the therapist has to let go and enable the person to activate the power to choose. At that point therapists could consider putting mechanisms in place to ensure the environment is as safe as possible. For example, a home visit might ensure the removal of area rugs, thus eliminating one potential cause of falls. Family members could be advised about volunteer community services that might offer assistance with tasks such as shopping. Follow-up home visits could be arranged for a few weeks hence to address problems that have arisen since discharge.

Therapist confidence

There are several reasons why therapist confidence is an important issue to consider before deciding to implement a client-centred approach. It has already been mentioned that it takes confidence to support a client's decision in the face of opposition from other team members. It also takes confidence to be certain that all the necessary information has been provided to the client in a way that was thoroughly understood before reaching a decision. Therapists must have confidence that their knowledge base is sound enough to support the information being given to the client. A professional's ability to solve problems gains strength from the application of scientific

theory and techniques (Schon 1983). Barriers arise if the therapist lacks either knowledge about client-centred practice or self-knowledge (Fraser 1995, Law et al 1995, Levenstein et al 1986). Self-knowledge ensures that the therapist is comfortable with personal boundaries and the reality of limited capabilities. Clients may want to establish goals that are quite unrealistic. It takes confidence to reassess the information given to the client that led to the establishment of that goal and to reframe the information for further review. Confidence is also attached to the ability to be flexible enough to meet the demands of individual clients. If therapists are going to facilitate client choice then they must be ready to work with choices that are different for each individual. Working in partnership with clients also requires the application of a range of skills from administration to politics and from teaching to being a mechanic. The confidence factor applies not only to acquiring and using these skills but also to knowing the depth of application that is required.

Other therapist components

There are many things that are part of a therapist's being and hence mould how he or she approaches work tasks. These include the therapist's values and beliefs, which must have an impact on how the tasks are performed. If the therapist believes that humans are innately strong, then expecting clients to cope with a wide range of adversities will guide the interventions that are suggested. On the other hand, if the belief system focuses on human weakness, then the expectations will have a different focus. Beliefs and values are complex but therapists must clearly understand their own and how they impact on their approach to clients. The therapist's personal values must also be separated from the professional ones, as well as from the client's values. This can be a particular challenge if the client is making a decision that the therapist views as unsafe (Law et al 1995).

The therapist's ability to build rapport will also have a major impact on the ability to adopt a client-centred approach. In order for clients to accept power they must trust the person who is assisting them with that responsibility. This development of trust begins at the first encounter and continues until the process comes to an end. If a positive rapport has been established the client will not fear asking questions, which is an essential ingredient in ensuring that information is understood. It is less difficult to ask what may appear to be an embarrassing or insignificant question if you have a meaningful relationship with the person who has the answers.

Other barriers that the therapist might bring to the encounter include ethical considerations, ability to access information and general communication skills. Is it ethical to refuse funding to help an elderly client who refuses to have bath rails installed because they will ruin the decor she has planned so carefully? The therapist knows that with these rails the client would be able to bath independently and safely. Without them she will be in serious danger of falling and will require expensive home help. Volumes have been written about ethics and ethical dilemmas, and the issues will not be resolved here. The point being made in this discussion is simply that the way a therapist views the ethics of the situation may prevent the application of a client-centred approach. The client has the right to refuse the bath rails but the therapist must have confidence that this decision was made following receipt and understanding of the relevant information.

The importance of the client having the information needed before making a decision has already been addressed. However, a barrier is created if the therapist is unable to access the necessary information. As this information relates to a wide range of client goals, some creative strategies may be required. In this age of rapidly expanding information it is unlikely that all the required resources will be located in the occupational therapy department. External sources such as medical and local libraries, community programmes and the World Wide Web will need to be used with increasing frequency. Therapists may be able to assist clients in accessing these sources of information rather than having to locate all the information themselves. The sharing of this responsibility enhances the strength of the partnership.

Communication skills have received attention in previous sections of this text. They are mentioned here to remind therapists that it is useless to collect high-quality information if the essence of it cannot be communicated effectively. Clients, significant others in their lives, and members of the occupational therapy and multidisciplinary teams must all receive this information in a manner that clearly establishes its relevance.

Other barriers that therapists might bring to the implementation of client-centred practice include high levels of stress (Ku 1993) created by unrealistic caseloads and performance expectations as well as ever-expanding knowledge that must be incorporated into current practice. Therapists may also view client-centred practice as too great a change from current practice (Stewart and Harvey 1990, Toomey et al 1995). Not everyone responds positively to change and the challenges presented by a change to client-centred practice may be insurmountable for some therapists. Issues also relate to the client and therapist being of different genders or cultures (Dyck 1989, Law and Britten 1995). There may be cultural reasons why a client-centred approach is not the appropriate one to use. However, conflict will result if either the therapist or client fails to recognise this concern. The therapist may also be concerned that client-centred practice is too demanding of the client (Koska 1990, Gage 1994). Generally client-centred practice does place greater demands on the client, which presents additional challenges to people dealing with problems. However, the challenge for the therapist is to present the approach at a level that facilitates the resolution of problems rather than adding to them.

Client barriers

The barriers that may be presented by the client fall into several categories. The first relates to social and family issues. Clients may traditionally have lacked power and are therefore in a position where they fear what will happen to them if they do not comply with someone else's wishes. They may be intimidated by hospital staff or professional people in general, and in the therapeutic environment will choose not to take responsibility for themselves.

Education may also be a barrier. Clients may lack an understanding of the rationale behind client-centred practice or the confidence that comes with advanced levels of education. They may lack previous opportunities to question information that is given to them and hence be reluctant to admit that they have not understood the presented material.

Cultural issues that were discussed in Chapter 3 in relation to the cultural environment may also pose barriers to the client taking full advantage of the intervention being client centred. The culture may encourage the maintenance of the sick role and the acceptance of how sick people perform. This performance may not include accepting the power to make decisions about the goals and means to accomplish them. Clients may also be expected to maintain a stiff upper lip and not to complain or disagree with the direction the intervention is taking. The client may see the professional as the expert and expect them to take a leading role and direct the intervention. The client may also simply be too ill or tired to expend the energy required in making decisions.

Problem-solving skills are required to participate fully in client-centred practice. When clients do not possess these skills, therapists may have to be more directive than would be their choice when attempting to implement client-centred practice (Law et al 1995). Additional client barriers presented by an elderly client group are discussed by Sandra Hobson in Chapter 7.

Barriers presented by the work environment

Time factor

There are many environmental pressures that affect the way therapists work including the pressure of time (Ku 1993). There is never enough time to do everything that needs to be done and employers are asking therapists to see an increasing number of clients in an attempt to decrease waiting lists and ensure ongoing funding. The rapid pace of this throughput places added stress on both the client and the therapist. From this perspective, client-centred practice does not appear to be a reasonable option. It does take more time to explain information in a style that is adapted for each individual and that is provided at the depth required for the client to make important decisions.

Therefore, if viewed over a short timespan, client-centred practice is more time consuming. This fact must be considered in the light of the increasing importance being placed on quality of care. This approach may take more time initially but it improves the quality of the service being provided to the client. However, in the long term, client-centred practice should be less time consuming as the client gains expertise in identifying issues of concern and in assuming responsibility for goals. If more time is spent initially in helping a client to understand the issues related to the problem and working in partnership to devise an intervention that the client owns, then less time is required to ensure that the programme is being followed and that the client is assuming responsibility for his own ongoing management.

Issues related to the multidisciplinary team

Client-centred practice works in harmony with other models and approaches. However, it is difficult for an occupational therapist to use a client-centred approach if the other members of the team follow a traditional approach and are more directive. Confusion will result for clients who are being advised by the occupational therapist that they can determine the goals for the intervention while being told by other team members what course of action to follow. Frustration will result for the therapist who wants to champion the client's chosen course of action but who knows that the decision will not be supported by other members of the team. This issue is very closely connected to the earlier discussion related to therapist confidence. It takes considerable courage to tackle a team in order to support a client's choice in the face of opposition which inevitably carries more power if only because of the number of people who are opposed.

Funding and philosophy

The financial priorities of the programme may not allow the flexibility of taking more time to help a client establish goals that are personally meaningful. There may not be the resources for the establishment of programmes that would truly meet the client's needs. If the programme is dominated by the medical model it may be difficult to implement client-centred practice (Crowe 1994, Johnson 1993). The key components of client-centred practice, such as autonomy and responsibility, do not fit with a system that insists on being staff led. Funding is usually directed toward the issues that are outlined in the philosophy of the programme and hence there are problems in securing funding for programmes that counter the favoured approach.

CONCLUSION

None of these obstacles is insurmountable but several may require creative problem-solving to remove them. It is clear from this discussion, as well as the preceding ones and those to follow, that it is neither simple nor easy to implement a client-centred approach. However, therapists must not lose sight of the reasons the programme exists and the importance of maintaining the focus on clients and the central position of their role in the process.

This chapter concludes the discussion of background information that it is necessary for the therapist to consider before implementing a client-centred approach. It is advisable for the reader to have considered the first four chapters before proceeding to read subsequent sections that focus on application.

REFERENCES

Canadian Association of Occupational Therapists 1991 Occupational therapy guidelines for client centred practice. CAOT Publications ACE, Toronto

Canadian Association of Occupational Therapists 1997 Enabling occupation: an occupational therapy perspective. CAOT Publications ACE, Toronto

Clemens E, Wetle T, Feltes M, Crabtree B, Dubitzky D 1994 Contradictions in case management. Journal of Aging and Health 6(1):70–88

College of Occupational Therapists 1995 Code of ethics and professional conduct for occupational therapists. College of Occupational Therapists, London

Crowe M 1994 Problem based learning: a model for graduate transition in nursing. Contemporary Nurse 3(3):105–109

Deber R B 1994 The patient physician partnership: changing roles and the desire for information. Canadian Medical Association Journal 15(2):171–176

Dyck I 1989 The immigrant client: issues in developing culturally sensitive practice. Canadian Journal of Occupational Therapy 56(5):248–255

Epstein R M, Campbell T L, Cohen-Cole S A, McWhinney I R, Smilkstein G 1993 Perspectives on patient doctor communication. Journal of Family Practice 37(4):377–388

Fraser D M 1995 Client centred care: fact or fiction? Midwives June:174–177

Gage M 1994 The patient driven interdisciplinary care plan. Journal of Nursing Administration 24(4):26–35

Gerhardt U 1989 Ideas about illness: an intellectual and political history of medical sociology. Macmillan, Basingstoke

Gustafson D 1991 Expanding the role of patient as consumer. Quality Review Bulletin October:324–325

Henderson A 1994 Power and knowledge in nursing practice: the contribution of Foucault. Journal of Advanced Nursing 20:935–939

Herzberg S R 1990 Client or patient: which term is more appropriate for use in occupational therapy? American Journal of Occupational Therapy 44(6):561–564

Hobson S 1996 Being client centred when the client is cognitively impaired. Canadian Journal of Occupational Therapy 63(2):133–137

Hokanson Hawks J 1991 Power: a concept analysis. Journal of Advanced Nursing 16:754–762

Johnson R 1993 Attitudes don't just hang in the air – disabled people's perceptions of physiotherapists. Physiotherapy 79(9):619–627

Kielhofner G 1985 A model of human occupation: theory and application. Williams and Wilkins, Baltimore

Koska M 1990 Patient centred care: can your hospital afford not to have it? Hospitals November:48–54

Ku K 1993 Life vs. death: client centred approach in nursing the dying children and their families. Hong Kong Nursing Journal 62(6):16–22

Law M, Baptiste S, Mills J 1995 Client-centred practice: what does it mean and does it make a difference? Canadian Journal of Occupational Therapy 62(5):250–257

Law S, Britten N 1995 Factors that influence the patient centredness of a consultation. British Journal of General Practice 45:520–524

Levenstein J H, McCracken E C, McWhinney I R, Stewart M, Brown J B 1986 The patient centred clinical method. 1. A model for the doctor patient interaction in family medicine. Family Practice 3(1):24–30

Mold J W, Blake G H, Becker L A 1991 Goal oriented medical care. Family Medicine 23(1):46–51

Raatikainen R 1994 Power or the lack of it in nursing care. Journal of Advanced Nursing 19:424–432

Reilly M 1984 The importance of the client versus patient issue for occupational therapy. American Journal of Occupational Therapy 38(6):404–406

Richards T 1998 Partnership with patients. British Medical Journal 316:85–86

Rogers C 1983 Freedom to learn for the 80's. Charles E Merrill, Columbus, Ohio

Schon D A 1983 The reflective practitioner: how professionals think in action. Basic Books, USA

Sharrott G W, Yerxa E J 1985 Promises to keep: implications of the referent patient versus client for those served by occupational therapy. American Journal of Occupational Therapy 39(6):401–405

Stewart D, Harvey S 1990 Application of the guidelines for client centred practice to paediatric occupational therapy. Canadian Journal of Occupational Therapy 57(2):88–94

Swaffield L (1990) Patient power. Nursing Times 86(48):26–28

Toomey M, Nicholson D, Carswell A 1995 The clinical utility of the Canadian Occupational Performance Measure. Canadian Journal of Occupational Therapy 62(5):242–249

5

Implementing
client-centred practice

D. M. Parker

Interpreting the philosophy of client centredness into
everyday practice requires a shift in the relationship
between client and therapist. This chapter advises
therapists, particularly managers, on how to make this
change by identifying the issues involved and adopting a
clear strategy for achievement. In doing so, it draws on
the author's own experience of implementing client-
centred practice in three distinct clinical areas.

INTRODUCTION

How comfortable are you with understanding
and using models of practice? Hands up those of
you who qualified over 10 years ago who confi-
dently came up with an answer. If this question
made you pause for thought, then read on…

Current students of the profession of occupational therapy are well versed in the art, and
science, of models, frames of reference and para-
digms. They can name names and explain structure, but can they put theory into practice? Can
you, as a manager, determine which model of
practice your therapists are using and can you
check that they are consistent?

It is all very well knowing your theory, but
if theory remains the domain of the academics
and is not tried out in the field, then it will
become stale and the profession will fail to
develop. Worse still, practice will be out of step
with current academic research and vice versa.

Implementing client-centred practice into the
workplace first of all requires a theoretical understanding of the philosophy of client centredness.
With this must come a belief in its efficacy;
in other words it must feel real to you as the

therapist. Interpreting this philosophy into every-day practice demands a fundamental shift in the way clients are approached and requires much debate and ongoing discussion to develop ideas and practice. Managing this change and ensuring smooth implementation can be achieved by identifying the issues involved and adopting a clear strategy for achievement.

This chapter addresses this process in a practical way, based on the experiences of implementing a client-centred approach within the National Health Service (NHS). The author has implemented client-centred practice into three distinct clinical areas; the process of implementation has involved learning from each situation and adapting to the unique circumstances of each area.

Clinical Area 1

Venue: A busy acute physical department, part of a major teaching hospital providing regional and supraregional specialties with a high level of medical expertise.

Occupational therapy team: Nine qualified staff with two support workers.

Beds: 500 inpatient beds.

Clinical field: Neurosciences, general medicine, acute elderly, oncology and transplantation programmes in heart, liver and kidney.

Unique features: The occupational therapy team members were a cohesive group. Each worked independently as part of a multidisciplinary team on their own ward areas. Liaison was important both internally with other therapists, ward staff and social work teams, and externally with community-based staff providing community care and discharge provision. Throughput was heavy with much emphasis on fast and efficient discharges.

Model of care: Medical model in the hospital.

Clinical Area 2
Venue: A hospice based in the community providing palliative care.

Occupational therapy team: a senior therapist and support worker.

Beds: 25 inpatient beds; outpatient and day care.

Clinical field: All conditions of adult oncology with some referrals from neurosciences.

Unique features: Occupational therapy staff were an integral part of the multidisciplinary team within the hospice. Patient and carer involvement was closely linked to therapeutic care.

Model of care: Client centred.

Clinical Area 3
Venue: Community residential rehabilitation centre.

Occupational therapy staff: Clinical specialist occupational therapist leads a therapy team of two occupational therapists, two physiotherapists and one technical instructor.

Beds: 22 residential rooms; two flats for independent living.

Clinical field: Acute physical and social rehabilitation programmes for medically stable disabled adults.

Unique features: This unit was established as a collaborative venture between health, social services, education and the voluntary sector to provide a holistic approach to rehabilitation.

Model of care: Client centred; the philosophy is based within the social model of rehabilitation.

Each of these areas has presented with its own difficulties and challenges in implementing client-centred practice and should supply the reader with some insight into the issues and solutions. They will be referred to throughout the chapter.

ISSUES IN IMPLEMENTING CLIENT-CENTRED PRACTICE
Staff-related issues

Making the decision

The wise manager is one who heeds the saying 'a fool and his words are soon parted' (Shenstone 1764), because client centredness is about practice and is not just a philosophy based on words.

Ideally there should have been some process by which the decision to adopt client-centred practice has been made. This process may be an internal one; for example, perhaps you as manager have decided to identify what model of practice your staff are using. Taking on new occupational therapy staff or students often raises interest in new approaches. The impetus for change may come about by sharing new ideas and innovations, or by challenging existing beliefs and knowledge.

Alternatively, the impetus for change may be external. For example, occupational therapy managers may be asked for outcomes of their service or may be required to explain why a particular intervention works and to identify the model of practice that is being used. In a health-care industry that reacts to external pressures, we as therapists need to be responsive to change. This change in approach may have been forced on the service as a result of political pressures. Health service strategies are often rife with trends in approaches and jargon which usually have a limited lifespan but which impact on service delivery. In the case of the writer, the impetus for change to a client-centred model of practice came about as a result of three significant factors occurring in Clinical Area 1.

First, the increasing pressure on the department to respond to the fast throughput of admissions meant that there was the threat of therapists becoming merely discharge coordinators with the resultant loss of core skills. This frustration with the medical model of practice led the therapy team to consider the roots of occupational therapy to identify a model of practice that better expressed how therapists worked.

Second, the department had worked hard at developing clinical and professional standards of practice and audit measures which were owned and used by the team. The next stage on from this was to consider outcomes of intervention.

Lastly, the manager had embarked on postgraduate study which involved detailed evaluation of the theories underpinning occupational therapy. The next logical step led the manager to use and evaluate a client-centred outcomes measure, a consequence of which was that the team adopted a client-centred approach within the department and found that it fulfilled their desire to work closer to their core skills.

Managers and therapists should be clear about terminology. They should not confuse client-centred practice with patient-focused care, and should not allow health service bosses to be confused about the differences between these approaches. It is the manager's responsibility to ensure that, if adopting the client-centred approach, then this is identifiable in practice.

Patient-focused care is clearly defined as 'the re-design of patient care so that hospital resources and personal care are organised around patients rather than around various specialised departments' (British Association of Occupational Therapists 1994). It is distinctly different to client-centred practice. Patient-focused care may be interpreted as 'management-speak' for patient coordinated care. The philosophical background and the emphasis in client-centred practice on the collaborative relationship with the client are two key areas of difference.

Alternatively, the manager may have identified a conscious shift in approach by the staff team away from the mechanistic reductionist medical model of practice to a more humanistic one. Others may have concluded that, as a result of clinical reasoning, client-centred practice was the only meaningful way forward. Sumsion (1993) supports the notion that client-centred practice is a greater challenge and that it provides a good example of where we can use our clinical reasoning skills.

The specific process used to reach the decision to implement a client-centred approach is perhaps less important than the acknowledgement that adopting a process that suits the working environment must be given careful consideration before the final decision is made. Once the decision has been made to adopt a client-centred approach, attention to the following issues will facilitate the implementation.

Compliance

The decision to adopt a client-centred approach must be endorsed by the occupational therapy team if it is to be implemented with success. Therefore the manager must ensure that the occupational therapy staff understand what client-centred practice means, and that they can apply the theory in practice. This will ensure consistency of approach and avoid inequality in client care.

Compliance is a conviction that should be tested in practice. In other words, therapists who say they are client centred and who then devise intervention plans to the exclusion of the client clearly require further exploration of their knowledge. Consider this example:

An occupational therapy team met to discuss and explore the merits and disadvantages of client-centred practice. All contributed their own ideas and definitions of the model in practice. In conclusion, all members of the team appeared to have grasped the theory of the approach and were keen to put theory into practice. In a review one month later it emerged that one therapist had had difficulty in doing so. She did not want to relinquish the responsibility of planning intervention. Involving the client in the goal setting and intervention planning meant, to her, that she had lost control. So, whilst this therapist agreed in theory, she had much more to learn and understand in practice about compliance with the client-centred approach.

Role model

In any departmental team, the effect and influence of role models should never be underestimated. Key senior staff exert considerable influence over juniors and students, and provide both positive and negative role models (Kielhofner 1992). This may be demonstrated overtly by means of practice observation, shadowing and teaching specific techniques, or covertly by influencing practice through supervision, support and objective setting. The influence of experience over naïveté

should be a reminder to any manager wishing to implement a new working practice that senior therapists need to endorse the new way forward or they may provide a negative role model for juniors.

Confidence

Any change in practice requires knowledge, understanding, debate, practice, feedback and confidence (Reilly 1984). How many departments can consciously identify their approach to patient care, specify the model and debate and practice it with fluency?

Confident readers who readily make time available for updating their knowledge, or who have recently qualified or pursued postgraduate education, may find this question somewhat irrelevant. Others, though, who do not have the luxury of recent qualification on their side, or who may not be supported in their endeavours to access study time, may find they are unable to answer this question. Whatever the response, the individual's ability to embrace a new way of working may challenge, threaten or stimulate their confidence. It is the manager's responsibility to establish the confidence levels of the staff team members if the intention is to implement a new working practice. If confidence is poor then steps need to be taken to improve it, or practice will be affected.

Suggestions for improving staff confidence
Teamworking Cohesion and support from the occupational therapy team will provide peer trust and good communication vital for implementing new approaches.

Case study: the need for a positive role model

An example of this need was seen with the use of the Canadian Occupational Performance Measure (COPM), a client-centred outcomes measure. Working within Clinical Area 1, a senior therapist claimed to be client centred. However, when it came to practising in a client-centred manner the senior therapist declined to use the COPM on the grounds that an elderly person would not understand how to score themselves. A junior therapist working with her found it so difficult to contradict her approach and maintain a working relationship with the senior that she adopted the same attitude. The senior therapist had problems grasping the real challenge of client-centred practice and proved a dominant role model for the junior.

Conversely, another senior therapist, who was working in Clinical Area 3 and was successfully adopting a client-centred approach, provided an excellent teaching opportunity, demonstrated sound practice and encouraged confidence in the skills of client centredness.

This positive role model can assist in the training and confidence-building of other staff.

Discussion and debate. Opportunities should be made for regular team reviews and meetings to explore new practice, developments and problems.

Reflective practice. Occupational therapy staff should try using a reflective practice diary to note problems, achievements and ways of tackling specific client-centred issues. These can then be used during supervision to illustrate particular points and reward individual achievements.

Case presentation. Once trust and teamwork have been established, regular case presentations can be used to explore difficult issues, to solve problems and to discuss approaches. Clarifying your approach and intervention with your peers can boost confidence and confirm standards of practice.

A study on the introduction of the COPM showed that low confidence levels in administering this measure was a significant factor in the poor uptake of the measure (Parker 1995). By contrast, those who felt more confident and who used the COPM more fluently demonstrated a greater practical awareness of client-centred practice. Confidence can be gained if practice is endorsed from the top. Teamworking can provide peer support, and supervision can be used to clarify performance and reward achievements. Confidence in being client centred will remain low if the safety net of peer support and supervision is removed and good practice is not applauded.

Occupational therapy team support

Implementing client-centred practice within an occupational therapy team demands time, effort and debate to establish a working understanding of the issues. Commitment needs to be given to this by individual team members in terms of both time and energy. Some team members may be reluctant to sacrifice valuable clinical time for other activities, especially if there is pressure on them to empty hospital beds.

Care should also be taken to ensure that therapists do not use the excuse of 'patients come first' to avoid new practice or updating skills. Others may be intimidated by more dominant members of the group who are forceful in their

views and are carried along with the philosophy but fail to deliver in practice.

Teamwork allows difficulties to be shared and strengths to be utilised. Individuals can be encouraged to support and work with others within the group, thus providing a focus for team building. Oakland (1989) places teamwork, involvement and problem-solving firmly within the context of successful quality management.

Team support can also assist in exploring difficult issues in client-centred practice such as cases of conflict. Consider this example:

In Clinical Area 1 a therapist is carrying out a client-centred programme and setting up the discharge for an elderly man for whom there will be risks at home. Conflict arises when the relatives decide the man should be placed in a nursing home to be cared for. The client is fully aware of the risks and is adamant about going home. The therapist has carried out a client-centred assessment and has identified the problems with the client and actioned solutions. Whilst the therapist feels sure she is acting in the client's best and expressed wishes, she is worried about the reaction of the relatives. She talks this over in supervision and agrees to the suggestion to present this case at the next team training session. The team discusses the case and supportively encourages the therapist to analyse her intervention, to act as the client's advocate and to prepare her argument in support of the client against the views of the relatives.

This is an example of the challenge a therapist may face when facilitating the shift in power to the client. Harnessing team support will ensure greater success in implementing client-centred practice.

Management support

There is no doubt that implementing any change in practice requires not only time and commitment from staff but also support and encouragement from occupational therapy and hospital management. This may take the form of approved study time or time out from clinical work for discussion and evaluation, or the provision of training facilities, for example purchase of the Self Instructional Package for the COPM*.

---

* The COPM Self Instructional Package is available from the Canadian Association of Occupational Therapists and the College of Occupational Therapists in England.

Provision of research opportunities to explore the theory and practice of client-centred practice may provide useful indicators of the measure of management support. Whatever the resource implications of instituting change, it is important to strike a balance between time spent in clinical work and that spent developing practice.

Practice-related issues

Conflict

Once the commitment has been made to adopt a client-centred approach, the next stage for planning is to determine how to put the approach into practice. Managers should be aware of the environment in which their teams function and the philosophical approach used, however indistinct this may be. Adopting client-centred practice may cause conflict for the staff with others who adopt a very different approach. The potential for conflict with other practice models has been discussed in earlier chapters.

Using a client-centred approach in Clinical Area 2 was relatively easy as the working environment (the hospice) was itself a model of client centredness.

The most common conflict in the work environment is likely to be a clash with the other models, particularly the medical model with its rather mechanistic, diagnosis-led approach which can ignore the individual in the bed. Conflict is most obvious in the acute sectors of the health service where pressure on beds and the urge to discharge challenge the role and purpose of occupational therapy (Blain and Townsend 1993).

In practice, many therapists consider that the main conflict between client-centred practice and the medical model remains an issue of control and timeliness of intervention rather than an overwhelming philosophical issue (Parker 1995).

Control and autonomy

Adopting a client-centred approach challenges the individual therapists to examine their own views of the client and the role they play in rehabilitation. As part of the therapist's own

learning and acceptance of the philosophy, the issues of control and advocacy need to be addressed.

The therapist who finds it easier to deliver a prescriptive programme of therapy is the one who prefers to retain control of the intervention. The move towards client autonomy may create conflict for the therapist who has the desire to care for others (Barnitt 1994). Failure to recognise the need for partnership with the client in intervention will jeopardise the implementation of client-centred practice. Whilst acknowledging that client-centred practice necessarily leads to a change in power relations, Law et al (1995) remind us that client and therapist become partners in the intervention process. The manager should endeavour to recognise the fear of loss of control and the real challenges that client-centred practice pose to a therapist. Support, supervision and training should be offered to therapists who find it hard to accept the client-centred approach. Managers should acknowledge that, just as clients are individual, therapists too are unique in their own way and may need to express client centredness within their own limitations. Better the fears that you know than the ones you have not exposed.

Greater skill is required to be client centred, to develop the relationship with the client within an often limited timeframe, to encourage empowerment and to deliver the intervention in partnership with the client, because this approach demands a recognition of the risks (Law et al 1994). Recognition of the change in role from a patient to that of a client needs to be explored, debated, understood and ultimately accepted if client-centred practice is to be adopted (Davidson 1991).

Intervention

Time and its influence on client-centred practice is an important issue in intervention. If insufficient time is spent on assimilating both the philosophy and the practice of client centredness, then confidence levels of the staff may suffer (Parker 1995). Knowledge and skills requirements change if a new approach is adopted, and the learner must change in response to this new and altered information (Reilly 1984). If a different approach is implemented without prior investment in learning then intervention will suffer as a result. Therapists may also ignore a new way forward in preference for an approach that provides expedient results, and one which they can practise with familiarity.

An additional impact of using a new technique is having the time to use it properly, especially when the demand to vacate beds and organise discharges is a constant pressure. This may affect the quality and standard of the service. Managers need to provide support to therapists struggling with a philosophy and approach that may place them in conflict with colleagues over intervention and discharge.

Therapists who fail to grasp the holistic nature of the client-centred approach may struggle with forming realistic intervention plans which truly reflect the client's expressed needs. Consider the case study from Clinical Area 1. In this example a therapist identifies risks of safety but the client has not identified any – and indeed denies there is a problem.

To approach this client-centredly, the therapist needs to agree a joint goal with Mrs A, who is desperate to go home whatever the problems. Next the therapist must determine with Mrs A what she needs to achieve in order to go home. Then she must identify with Mrs A what actions can be taken to reduce the risks to ensure a safe discharge. The following actions were taken:

• A second stair rail was fitted.
• The stair carpet was secured.

• The physiotherapist gave Mrs A extra practice at stairs, concentrating on how to pace herself.
• Mrs A agreed to a commode downstairs as long as her granddaughter was the only one to empty it.
• Mrs A practised using a trolley to help with meal preparation.
• Her granddaughter did her shopping, but Mrs A prepared the list, which now included precooked meals for reheating in a new microwave oven.
• Community transport was arranged for trips to the bingo club.

The way forward for the therapist is to appreciate the need to develop a partnership approach with the client and ensure ownership of the issues rather than take control and alienate the client, thus straying from client centredness.

Some clients will undoubtedly have limited insight into their problems and circumstances, for example those with brain injury, cognitive dysfunction or degenerative (Alzheimer) disease. However, it is the quality of the approach that is all important. A therapist can still be client centred when working with clients with limited insight, purely by ensuring their involvement in the intervention process, rather than removing that control entirely. Hobson (1996) suggests exploring the techniques of graded decision making and advocacy as two methods for practising in a client-centred manner with cognitively impaired clients.

Case study from Clinical Area 1

Mrs A is a 62-year-old woman with chronic renal failure which has contributed towards a gradually dependent lifestyle over recent years. She lives alone in her own house and has one daughter who lives nearby but who is unable to provide any daytime help as she works full time. The daughter is concerned for her mother's safety on discharge and wonders whether she can really cope, especially as several burnt cooking pots have been discovered and she suspects her mother leaves the gas on.

A granddaughter has a very close relationship with Mrs A; they appear to understand each other well, and she is keen to help Mrs A once discharged home.

Using the COPM, Mrs A has expressed problems with her walking, especially in negotiating the stairs. The physiotherapist has assessed her as unsafe on the stairs as she tends to rush. Other occupational performance problems include organising her own meals, shopping, getting to the bingo club and exercising her dog. The therapist is concerned that Mrs A fails to realise how unsafe she is on the stairs and has tried to encourage her to sleep downstairs, which she refuses to do.

Case study from Clinical Area 3

Mr B is 25 years old and sustained a head injury in an accident at work. Whilst he has regained full mobility, he has a tendency to fall when tired or if he rushes about. He has expressive speech problems and some cognitive dysfunction, especially with regard to motor relearning. Mr B is very keen to learn how to do more in the house, especially making his own meals and getting out to meet his friends. He has agreed to return to live with his family, but his parents are anxious about leaving him home alone as they are at work during the day.

The therapist completes a COPM with him and identifies some occupational performance problems, but due to his lack of insight and cognitive problems Mr B fails to understand the real depth of his difficulties. Involving him in the assessment process and completing a COPM with his parents present has allowed the therapist greater insight into his needs. The intervention plan included the introduction of a community service volunteer to work exclusively with him at home to ensure safety with household tasks and social rehabilitation.

Case study from Clinical Area 3

Mr C is a 46-year-old sales-person admitted for further rehabilitation. He sustained spinal injuries as a result of a road traffic accident and consequently is now paraplegic. He is determined to lead a completely independent lifestyle and resents help or interference. As part of his assessment he has expressed having some difficulty with his transfers, especially in and out of his car and into the bath. The therapist assesses his function and suggests an alternative method of transferring. Mr C does not agree with this method and demonstrates his own unique, if somewhat bizarre, method.

Consider the case study of Mr B from Clinical Area 3. Here the therapist may have to take greater initiative in planning and identifying problems but should endeavour to include the client in the process throughout.

Chapters 6 and 7 provide more detailed discussion of the issues to consider when working with this client group. Issues of client safety are commonly raised when the client-centred approach is used, especially in relation to those who have little or no insight (Law et al 1994).

The final case study of Mr C from Clinical Area 3 highlights the importance of focusing on the client's wishes.

The client-centred therapist is one who works with Mr C to reduce any risks involved in his transfers rather than insisting on him using the therapist's technique. Teaching him to understand the need for good skin care, weight transference and safe movement is far more important and client centred than insisting on a method that he will not use and ignoring

the method he has chosen. Again, client-centred practice is all about building the relationship between therapist and client, establishing good communication and trust, and encouraging understanding and insight.

Standards

If client-centred practice is to be adopted then this philosophy should be reflected in departmental standards which structure the quality of the practice. There should be a clear statement, endorsed by staff practice, which reflects the client-centred approach throughout intervention, treatment planning, discharge planning and follow-up.

Clear expectations of staff performance in terms of this approach can be built into professional standards, for example:

- 'All case notes will have a clear statement of client-centred goals.'
- 'All case notes will contain a written statement of client compliance with intervention.'

This can be monitored by clinical audit or service evaluation.

STRATEGIES FOR IMPLEMENTING CLIENT-CENTRED PRACTICE

Once the decision has been made to implement client-centred practice, the manager must decide how this is going to be achieved. This section deals with the practical realities of operating a client-centred philosophy based on the experience of implementing the COPM within an acute hospital, a hospice and a rehabilitation unit. It also considers why this approach has been implemented.

Ideas and strategies are put forward from personal experience within a particular NHS Trust; these may not be the solution for everyone. They may help you to develop a greater understanding of the team, stimulate individual debate and growth, and perhaps provide a trigger for your own ideas.

Education and training

First of all, know your staff. This may sound obvious but knowing their strengths, weaknesses, interests and skills will help to establish a clear profile of your workforce. It will help you, the manager, to identify resource issues, training needs, extra support and eliminate problem areas.

Ensure that supervision, both clinical and professional, is a regular feature for all therapists. This will enable weaknesses and problems to be dealt with individually. Supervision spread throughout all levels can also build support networks within the team itself. Obviously records of supervision must be kept, and individual staff members should also be encouraged to do so.

Link work objectives to enhance individual strengths and improve on problem areas. Also make sure that departmental objectives are reflected in individual work targets to ensure greater ownership and compliance with departmental development. If client-centred practice is to be adopted, then identify clearly with each staff member their role in this implementation and define how they can contribute by specifying this in their objectives.

Regular appraisal or individual performance review will similarly help to support and identify skills and strengths. Clarifying achievement of objectives and exploring the individual development of the client-centred philosophy will help individuals to recognise that they have a role within this implementation. Feedback on performance is vital for personal and professional growth.

Development of skills profiling to establish confidence levels can indicate training needs and expertise. A skills profile comprises a range of skills from clinical, professional, technical and personal which should reflect the wide range of tasks expected of therapists within the therapy team. Each skill can then be scored according to how confident each therapist considers he or she is in practice at each skill. This method enables the manager and the individual therapist to have a numerical confidence score across a wide range of skills, which may change over time. It affords the manager greater insight into the individual perception of confidence at occupational therapy tasks, and helps to identify training and support needs.

Recognition of the core skills of each grade of therapist throughout the team will ensure the correct skill mix and identify gaps and resources within the workforce.

Team building is imperative if a new philosophy is to be introduced which will affect practice. This can be achieved by training 'away days' on aspects of client-centred practice with an agreed action plan, timed implementation programme and named key personnel. Team building should also incorporate regular review sessions to monitor progress, determine difficult issues, and formulate and agree a way forward.

Another aspect of team building is to set up a system of mentors. These are senior practitioners who can support and develop the work of other staff members but who may not be directly responsible for their work. This has the further advantage of developing communication networks and trust throughout the team.

Use of mini pilot studies to work at particular issues can sharpen practice of new skills, maximise precious time and eliminate problems earlier, as well as drawing the team together. For example, in Clinical Area 2 staff had great reservations about using a client-centred outcomes measure within oncology. It was not so much a question of being client centred but more an issue of using an outcomes measure with those for whom life expectancy was limited. As a consequence staff were reluctant to use the COPM and expressed these fears openly. With encouragement from the medical director of the hospice, the COPM was used to determine some outcome measures within palliative care. A mini pilot study of short duration was carried out. Clients were assessed using the COPM and their feedback on this measure was documented. The senior therapist made a judgement on using the COPM based on the individual client's condition, mental state and degree of intrusion. Feedback gained from clients indicated a positive approval of involvement within the process of assessment, especially with regard to the empowerment of the client in the selection of goals, however limited these might have been. Use of this client-centred outcomes measure also gave the therapy staff very positive feedback on their role, in a clinical area where 'success' is compounded by death. Support from the other staff within the hospice meant that the introduction of client centredness was relatively easy.

Resources should also be identified to support training and education. This is not just about attending courses. Visits by staff to other centres or departments that have adopted a client-centred approach can boost an understanding of the issues in practice. Shadowing staff within the team who have already developed skills and expertise in client centredness will help to create positive role models.

Investment in training materials for home or 'in-house' study can similarly boost expertise and confidence. For example, the Self Instructional Programme for the COPM can be used by the team as a group training exercise. If cost is an issue here, then perhaps a copy shared across organisations is an option. Alternatively training sessions by experienced COPM users or client-centred practitioners can raise awareness, increase knowledge and confidence, and share skills. Training sessions can also be used to explore client-centred problems.

Networking through the profession may also identify departments with similar structures and services, where sharing knowledge can help to cut corners and develop ideas. Since studying the COPM, the writer has been contacted by other therapists interested in its use. As a result, a COPM network has been established to coordinate all those therapists across the UK who are using, who want to use, or who are thinking about using this outcomes measure. In this way skills can be shared, problems discussed and resolved and, most importantly, additions made to the body of knowledge of the profession. It has also provided the springboard for workshops to be held on the COPM.

Practice

Being client centred means putting your knowledge of the approach into practice, learning, developing and receiving feedback on that practice. Practical ways of achieving this include the following:

- Display a visual representation of the model on noticeboards and in clinical files. Fortunately the Model of Occupational Performance on which client-centred practice is based has an excellent diagram which clearly represents the model (Canadian Association of Occupational Therapists 1991) (see Ch. 1).
- Develop client-centred practice as a working philosophy expressed in all areas of contact with the client. For example, check that the department, the service and any marketing literature are client centred and friendly.
- Review all paperwork and forms to reflect a client-centred approach and ensure that forms are completed with the client. If resources permit, then self-duplicating assessment forms or intervention summaries would allow clients greater ownership, control and compliance by having access to information on their treatment. In Clinical Area 3 all clients hold their own copy of the COPM.
- Prepare a dossier of literature on client-centred practice and related subjects for each staff member, or develop a resource file on articles and contacts.
- Set up a simple log book for each staff member to document success and problems in their forays into client-centred practice. Staff can then use the examples in the log books to present as short problem scenarios to the team. This will improve presentation

skills, encourage communication of problems and achievements, and assist in boosting confidence.

- Case note audit and team audit of standards can similarly monitor practice and detect changes in approach towards client-centred practice. In Clinical Area 1 the team decided, as a result of their peer audit of case records, that they wanted a positive statement on client agreement to intervention included in the audit checklist.

- Develop interviewing skills by use of case studies and video feedback of practice interviews. Encourage the critique and evaluation of staff members' interviews to establish a standard in interviewing. Again in Clinical Area 1, staff requested feedback on interviewing skills as their confidence needed boosting in carrying out client-centred interviews.

- Use the Self Instructional Programme for the COPM which includes a video and notebook. This encourages close observation and critical analysis of various client-centred interviews, which can act as a fine teaching and learning tool.

- Establish the evaluation of outcomes within the department. Use of the COPM will ensure that the client-centred approach is used. Analysis of its administration may also highlight difficulties with client-centred practice.

- Provide feedback to the staff team on the change in practice either by encouraging self-evaluation of performance or by the analysis of outcomes data, complaints or compliments about the service. Feedback can also be given individually through supervision and appraisal.

- Encourage client feedback about the service with questions directed at eliciting an evaluation of the approach used by your staff. This might be achieved by phone or postal questionnaire, or by targeting specific client groups within the service and carrying out evaluative interviews. In Clinical Area 3 follow-up interviews are taking place six months after discharge to evaluate

consolidation of skills. Part of that evaluation is to reassess all occupational performance problems on the COPM and to gather client feedback on how a client-centred service has been delivered.

Finally, the question must be considered, why use this approach? Please do not just take my word for it: you must go out there and consider all the options for yourself. You know your own unique staff team, the demands and constraints on your service, and the resources available to you. You must make that decision.

There is no doubt that being client centred is challenging. It demands a high level of commitment, time and training. Staff need to be good 'people therapists' who can interview effectively and efficiently, and help clients to identify their goals. For clients who struggle with the responsibility of making choices about their future, the therapist needs to exercise sensitivity and clarity in order to empower them. With other clients who have problems of insight or intellect, the therapist needs to maintain their involvement whilst not losing sight of the goal.

Client-centred practice, however, does have definite advantages, not least because by following this approach we are adhering to the standards set by the professional bodies of occupational therapy, the College of Occupational Therapists in the UK and the Canadian Association of Occupational Therapists, to name but two. There is evidence in the literature that development of a client–therapist partnership can lead to increased client participation, client self-efficacy and improved satisfaction with the service. It is an approach that promotes respect for the partnership between therapists and clients (Law et al 1995).

Instead of promoting the manager's line about the need to adopt client-centred practice as the model for occupational therapy, the last comments come from the staff because, at the end of the day, they are the ones who will implement it.

In Clinical Area 1, one member of staff remarked that using the client-centred approach made greater sense of what she was trying to do, despite the constraints of time.

Action Checklist for Implementing Client-Centred Practice

1. Evaluate existing practice and attitudes.
2. Debate, discuss and explore issues with the team.
3. Educate, read and observe practice.
4. Provide support, supervision and training.
5. Develop a plan of action, pilot studies and trial interviews.
6. Implement client-centred practice into all aspects of assessment and intervention.
7. Review record-keeping.
8. Evaluate, audit and give feedback.

In Clinical Area 2, a senior therapist expressed her fears about using the COPM with the terminally ill. Once she had practised her interviewing skills she realised that being client centred brought the client's goals sharply into focus and made her job easier. She felt she was doing exactly what the client wanted and needed. Being client centred in a hospice was a lot easier because of their flexible approach.

Finally, in Clinical Area 3, a junior therapist who initially felt overwhelmed in her first real experience of a client-centred environment concluded that this approach was what occupational therapy was all about.

CONCLUSION

This chapter has described many of the issues facing a manager when considering the implementation of a client-centred approach both from a staff and from a practice point of view. The manager needs to empower and encourage the development of the team in order to achieve this goal. Practical strategies are suggested but they are not an exhaustive list. If managers are to demonstrate their own leadership skills then they must base their strategy for client-centred practice on their unique knowledge and understanding of their team and the constraints and opportunities facing their service. Managers must have their own vision.

REFERENCES

Barnitt R 1994 Patient agreement to treatment: a framework for therapists. British Journal of Therapy and Rehabilitation 1:3–4

Blain J, Townsend E 1993 Occupational therapy guidelines for client centred practice: impact study findings. Canadian Journal of Occupational Therapy 60(5):271–285

British Association of Occupational Therapists 1994 Patient focused care guidance for BAOT members. College of Occupational Therapists, London

Canadian Association of Occupational Therapy 1991 Guidelines for the client centred practice of occupational therapy. CAOT publications ACE, Toronto

Davidson H 1991 Performance and the social environment. In: Christiansen C, Baum C (eds) Occupational therapy; overcoming human performance deficits. Slack, Thorofare, New Jersey, pp 144–177

Hobson S 1996 Reflections on being client centred when the client is cognitively impaired. Canadian Journal of Occupational Therapy 63(2):133–136

Kielhofner G 1992 Conceptual foundations of occupational therapy. F A Davis, Philadelphia

Law M, Baptiste S, Carswell-Opzoomer A et al 1994 Canadian Occupational Performance Measure, 2nd edn. CAOT Publications ACE, Toronto

Law M, Baptiste S, Mills J 1995 Client centred practice: what does it mean and does it make a difference? Canadian Journal of Occupational Therapy 62(5):250–257

Oakland JS 1989 Total quality management. Butterworth-Heinemann, Oxford

Parker D 1995 An evaluation of the Canadian Occupational Performance Measure. MSc thesis, Exeter University

Reilly M 1984 The importance of the client versus patient issue for occupational therapy. American Journal of Occupational Therapy 38(6):404–406

Shenstone W 1764 On reserve. In: The concise Oxford dictionary of quotations, 3rd edn, vol 2. Oxford University Press, Oxford

Sumsion T 1993 Client centred practice: the true impact. Canadian Journal of Occupational Therapy 60(1):6–8

6

Using a client-centred approach with persons with cognitive impairment

S. J. G. Hobson

Clients with cognitive impairment are vulnerable to having their capacity to participate in client-centred care questioned. This chapter proposes that, despite barriers, it is possible to use this approach with these clients. Four specific strategies for client-centred care with this population will be described.

Occupational therapists regularly work with clients who have cognitive impairment. This can be temporary or persistent in nature. Temporary cognitive impairment may be associated with acute illness or medication side-effects. Persistent cognitive impairment may be secondary to a number of different diagnoses, including acquired brain injury, cerebral vascular accident, developmental delay, psychiatric illness and dementia of one sort or another. This chapter is primarily concerned with the issue of persistent cognitive impairment, although the strategies identified may work equally well for clients with temporary problems.

The exact prevalence of cognitive impairment is very difficult to estimate, given its multiple causes. However, recent statistics give hints of the scope of the issue. In the UK, dementia affects 650 000 individuals (Alzheimer's Disease Society 1998), traumatic brain injury affects 200 000 (Giles & Clark-Wilson 1993) and schizophrenia a further 250 000 (National Schizophrenia Fellowship 1998). In Canada, 'over 1 million adults have intellectual disabilities, learning disabilities or mental health conditions' (Statistics Canada 1994, p. xx), including 252 600 with dementia (Canadian Study of Health and Aging

Working Group 1994) and 83 000 with a mental handicap (Statistics Canada 1986). This totals over one million people in each country, with many causes of cognitive impairment not included.

But exactly what is meant by cognitive impairment? Cognition is defined as 'the mental process by which knowledge is acquired' and includes 'awareness ... perception, reasoning, judgement, intuition, and memory' (Thomas 1997, p. 408). Zoltan (1990) explained: 'Cognition allows individuals to use and process the information perceived to think and act' (p. 202). Obviously, impairment in any or all cognitive functions will seriously affect occupational engagement, making individuals with such impairments prime candidates for occupational therapy.

It seems clear, given the prevalence of such impairments, their impact on occupational performance and the fact that these impairments span the life course, that most occupational therapists will work with clients with cognitive impairment at some point in their careers. But is it possible to practise client-centred occupational therapy with these individuals? It has certainly been argued that a client with impaired reasoning, judgement and memory, all cognitive skills listed in the definition of cognition, would not be capable of establishing treatment goals and priorities or making treatment decisions. For example, Law et al (1995) specifically mention the client with poor problem-solving skills when discussing the challenges to implementing client-centred care.

This chapter will outline the counter-argument, that client-centred practice is possible, although not necessarily easy, with individuals with cognitive impairment. It will first consider the issue of capacity to participate in client-centred care, with special attention to elements considered most problematic, and then proceed to outline four specific strategies that therapists can use to assist in implementing client-centred care with these clients. These strategies include enhanced client assessment, graded decision-making, advocacy and surrogate client-centredness. Some of the ideas included in this chapter have been published previously (Hobson 1996).

CAPACITY TO PARTICIPATE IN CLIENT-CENTRED CARE

The earliest discussions of client-centred practice addressed the need for clients to have an active role in dealing with their problems 'without any notion of surrendering ... responsibility for the situation' (Rogers 1951, p. 7). Client involvement in defining programme goals, methods (Canadian Association of Occupational Therapists (CAOT) 1991) and the desired outcomes of therapy (Law et al 1995) is integral to client-centred practice.

The Canadian Occupational Performance Measure (COPM) was developed as 'an outcome measure for occupational performance' (Law et al 1991, p. 5) and is client centred in that it 'supports the notion that clients are responsible for their health and therapeutic process' (Law et al 1991, p. 10). Many occupational therapists have found the COPM helpful in initiating a client-centred relationship, because it solicits client involvement in establishing the goals and outcome measures for occupational therapy treatment. Despite the claim that it 'can be used across all developmental levels [and] can be used with all disability groups' (Law et al 1991, p. 10), the authors and others suggest that it may not be suitable for use with all client groups. Specifically mentioned as not suited to participation in the COPM are children, clients with cognitive impairment and those with psychiatric illness (Law et al 1995, Toomey et al 1995, Waters 1995). If the COPM is truely 'an excellent example of the application of the essence of the client-centred approach' (Sumsion 1993), but its use is questioned with clients with cognitive impairment, the feasibility of using a client-centred approach with these clients is called into question.

Informed consent to treatment is considered a first step in client-centred care (CAOT 1991). For consent to be informed, the individual must receive information on the alternative courses of treatment; the anticipated risks, benefits and side-effects of each potential course of treatment; and the consequences of not having any treatment at all (Ontario Ministry of Health 1994). Decision-making at subsequent stages in client-centred care, including therapeutic goal setting and the selection of treatment methods and desired outcomes, requires insight and judgement.

Venesy (1994) outlines the abilities required for competent decision-making as follows:

- The person is aware that there is a decision to be made, willing to make it, and able to communicate his or her decision.
- The person is able to understand the information necessary to make the decision, including the options available, pros and cons of each option, causal relationships, potential outcomes of each option, and the fact that the matter is personal to him or her, not merely abstract.
- The person's decision is stable over time and consistent with personal values.

The cognitive demands implicit in client-centred care are significant. In fact, it is considered an advanced form of clinical reasoning, conditional reasoning, for the therapist to project a realistic anticipated future for a given client (Fleming 1991). It is therefore understandable that questions are often raised about the ability of a client with cognitive impairment to participate in this sophisticated form of decision-making.

Competence is both a medically and a legally defined construct. In the literature the term capacity is sometimes used in lieu of competence. For clarity, in this chapter the term capacity will be used to refer to the medical construct, competence to refer to the legal one. Medical capacity refers to an individual's 'ability to perform mentally' (Thomas 1997, p. 299–300). Legal competence refers to 'being able to manage one's affairs, and by inference, being sane' (Thomas 1997, p. 424).

It is important to understand that these constructs, although related, are not identical. Not all individuals who are clinically deemed incapable have been declared legally incompetent; similarly, not all individuals who have been declared legally incompetent are medically incapable. This is partially because 'defining competence may be a little like defining obscenity; it eludes definition' (Jocobellis v Ohio 1964, as cited in Venesy 1994, p. 219). Further, current literature (Fulbrook

1994, Silberfeld 1992, Venesy 1994) and law (Bill 109 1992) on competence indicate that it is situational and is subject to change over time and under different circumstances (Venesy 1994). For example, a memory impairment may appear worse at the end of the day when compounded by fatigue, giving the health-care professional an exaggerated impression of client incompetence.

Thus far, the discussion has focused on the medical capacity of clients to participate in client-centred care, their ability to appreciate their own state of health, to understand the information about treatment options, and to remember it and manipulate it to form a reasoned decision. Client-centred care may be further complicated when individuals receiving the services have been deemed legally incompetent. In this case, they may not legally be permitted to give consent for the treatment, or they may not control their funds and, thus, may be unable to authorise the purchase of equipment or services required for implementation of the therapeutic plan. Under these circumstances, some other individual or organisation will have been appointed as substitute decision-maker for the client.

STRATEGIES FOR CLIENT-CENTRED CARE WITH PERSONS WITH COGNITIVE IMPAIRMENT

Despite the many difficulties identified above, there are four specific strategies that may assist the therapist in implementing client-centred care with persons with cognitive impairment. These strategies include enhanced client assessment, graded decision-making, advocacy, and surrogate client-centredness. These strategies will be discussed in turn.

Enhanced client assessment

Occupational therapy practice has been described as including seven steps: referral, assessment, programme planning, intervention, discharge, follow-up and programme evaluation (CAOT 1991). During the assessment phase, the client with cognitive impairment may have difficulty providing a detailed and accurate history. This is important if the therapy offered is to be contextually congruent (i.e. consistent with roles, interests, environments, culture and values), a feature that Law et al (1995) identify as a key element in client-centred care. Two specific suggestions will be made to enhance the assessment process for a client with cognitive impairment. These are clinical capacity assessment and extended history-taking.

Clinical capacity assessment

Occupational therapists may be involved in assessing capacity and/or competence. Regulations governing the assessment of legal competence vary according to jurisdiction. Because of the profound consequences of such a determination, the authority to declare someone incompetent is usually restricted to physicians. (Of interest, in Ontario, Canada, occupational therapists are among the five regulated health professions authorised to assess legal competence. The other professions include physicians and surgeons, psychologists, social workers and nurses (Ontario Ministry of the Attorney General 1996a).) It is important to recognise, however, that occupational therapists are frequently asked to comment on cognitive ability. Cognitive assessment and treatment are within occupational therapy's scope of practice, and physicians and others may request occupational therapy input when determining a client's legal competence. In many jurisdictions, the law is very non-specific about competence in cases other than psychiatric illness, and cognitive assessment results from an occupational therapist may be used to assist in substantiating a legal determination of incompetence for clients with cognitive impairment.

On the other hand, determination of medical capacity is an inherent part of clinical practice. In the words of Appelbaum and Grisso (1988): 'ordinarily the assessment of a patient's decision-making capacity is an implicit part of the doctor–patient interaction, often taking place without either party's awareness' (p. 1635). In practising client-centred care, the occupational therapist should be assessing the client's capacity to give informed consent at each decision point in the process. When assessing medical capacity, occupational therapists may benefit from the 'sliding scale' model (Venesy 1994, p. 220), whereby capacity is considered in relation to the potential consequences of the decision. If the risk associated with a decision is low, capacity need not be scrutinised too stringently, whereas when the risk is high capacity would be much more rigorously assessed. Many decisions associated with occupational therapy, such as a preferred treatment modality, would be low-risk decisions. Other decisions, such as discharge to an unsupervised living environment, would warrant very careful assessment of the client's medical capacity to recognise the risks inherent to each option under consideration and make a reasoned decision.

Venesy (1994) provides a clear outline of the basic requirements for making an informed decision. These were discussed earlier in this chapter and can be used to assess a client's medical capacity. Her requirements are congruent with the assessment for legal competence in Ontario, where the test addresses: (1) an individual's factual knowledge of (or ability to learn) the information needed to make a particular decision; (2) his or her awareness of options surrounding a decision; (3) his or her ability to appraise the potential outcome of a decision; and (4) his or her ability to explain some reasoned (NB this is differentiated from reasonable) justification for the decision (Ontario Ministry of the Attorney General 1996b). This is sometimes referred to as the 'understand and appreciate' test. It could also be used to assess a client's medical capacity.

Extended history-taking

During the assessment process, as noted earlier, the client with cognitive impairment may have difficulty providing a comprehensive and coherent history. If this is the case, additional efforts will have to be made to obtain detailed background information about a client. As indicated, this background is important so that the therapist can offer the client a suitable range of options from which to make choices. If the client has had a life-long interest in gardening, for instance, a horticulture programme may be a more suitable therapeutic activity than playing adapted checkers. This is particularly important when allied with graded decision-making, to be discussed next.

Extensive knowledge about the client can also assist the therapist to interpret the client's wishes more accurately, especially when the expression of these is equivocal or difficult to understand. An example of this, with which many therapists are familiar, is the failure to report pain in an effort to be a 'good patient' who is seen as compliant and/or cooperative. Those close to the client may be able to advise the therapist of other indicators of discomfort, such as becoming unusually withdrawn or quiet. Highly idiosyncratic use of certain colloquial expressions may be particularly difficult for therapists to understand fully. For example, the word 'tolerable' is a term of high praise for a friend of mine. Someone who did not know her well would very likely misinterpret her use of this word, assuming she intended the customary meaning of 'barely acceptable'.

Law et al (1995) state that respect for diversity, sometimes called culturally sensitive care (Anderson et al 1990), is an important part of client-centred care. Clients with cognitive impairment may be unable to explain cultural values and needs, but they may still respond negatively to any breech of cultural ethics, however inadvertent. Simple things like touching the head (Dihn et al 1990, Richardson 1990) or making direct eye contact (Lai & Yue 1990, Okabe et al 1990) may be intrusive or insulting to clients of come cultures. Even knowing the mores of a particular cultural group may not be sufficient, as individual members of a culture do not necessarily subscribe to all its values (Anderson et al 1990). The therapist can learn from significant others which particular cultural values the client may have held dear and, thus, avoid giving unintentional offence.

Family members and close friends can offer this type of background information about a client, and they are usually pleased to be asked

to do so. They are gratified to see such interest in the client as an individual. It is important to note that it may be necessary to gather information from several sources. This is particularly true when there is no consistent and/or long-standing companion available, such as a spouse.

Graded decision-making

Occupational therapists pride themselves on their skills in activity analysis, grading and adaptation. That is, they are skilled at assessing the physical, affective and cognitive demands of various activities, modifying the activity to match clients' abilities and/or adapting the activity to accommodate clients' disabilities. These skills can be applied to the task of decision-making. Decisions can be graded in a number of ways to allow clients of various levels of cognitive ability to succeed. A decision's cognitive demands can be modified by providing a *structure*. For example, the therapist could simplify the process by suggesting the client contrast pros, cons and probable outcomes of alternative decisions or by establishing a series of questions to be answered with regard to each option being considered. The therapist could create a *framework* for decision-making; that is, the client could be offered choice from within a set range of options. The framework could be expanded or contracted to offer as many options as the client was expected to be able to handle. The therapist could break the decision into a set of sequenced *steps*, such as selecting the desired or necessary features and identifying the affordable price range for a piece of equipment before selecting the preferred brand and colour. Offering clients choices appropriate to their cognitive ability is simply another form of determining the 'just right challenge' (Yerxa et al 1989, p. 12).

Even when a client has been deemed legally incompetent to make major decisions, it is both reasonable and possible to consult the client on specific aspects of care. Capacity is not a global construct; that is, people may be capable of making some decisions and not others (Fulbrook 1994, Silberfeld 1992, Venesy 1994). A client who may be incapable of consenting to a full course of treatment may be quite capable of expressing personal preferences about some element(s) of the course of treatment, which can be incorporated into the treatment plan. For example, a client experiencing postsurgical confusion may not be able to consent to the overall course of treatment for a hip fracture and replacement, but may be quite capable of expressing a preference for playing shuffleboard rather than bean bag toss while trying to increase standing tolerance.

The term 'client centred' has been criticised as too non-specific. In the words of Gage and Polatajko (1995): 'client-centred practice has been described as everything from considering the client's needs when making treatment decisions to having the client direct the care planning process' (p. 116). Gage and Polatajko view this as a limitation and advocate the use of the term 'client driven' to describe practice. The term 'client-centred', however, serves therapists practising with clients with cognitive impairment well precisely because it does recognize a variety of potential ways of interacting with clients. It might be inappropriate to practise client-driven occupational therapy with a client with cognitive impairment, but therapists should find it quite possible to practise client-centred occupational therapy with such clients.

Advocacy

Occupational therapists often work in teams in which not all professionals subscribe to client-centred principles, and they are accustomed to advocating on behalf of their clients. Advocacy is especially relevant when competence is called into question, because conformity is known to play a large role in competence decisions (Fiesta 1992, Venesy 1994). 'The question of competence is rarely raised unless there is an issue of non-compliance' (Fulbrook 1994, p. 458) with medical advice. Other pre-eminent risk factors for being declared incompetent include being among those who are 'elderly, mentally ill and mentally retarded adults, [and] head injured patients' (Venesy 1994, p. 219; see also Curtin 1995). The very fact of having a cognitive impairment may

put a client at risk of being treated as if he or she were incompetent, with no formal assessment whatsoever. Occupational therapists must ensure that their clients are not being summarily and inappropriately deprived of their right to consent to or to refuse treatment.

Advocacy is equally important when working with a client who has been found legally incompetent. In these cases, it is the occupational therapist's role to advocate for the client's wishes with the person who holds the legal authority to make treatment decisions. This means that therapists may risk being accused of introducing irrelevant information into the decision-making process, but they must have the courage to hold to their convictions regarding client-centred practice.

Another role for occupational therapists is to request and/or initiate reassessment of competence when they believe that the situation warrants it. It is acknowledged that 'competence may … fluctuate as a function of mood, time of day, metabolic status, pain, intercurrent illness or the effect of medication' (Venesy 1994, p. 222). Given that competence is increasingly defined as situation specific, clients have the right to make any decision for which they can give informed consent, at the moment that they can give it. The central precepts of informed consent are that 'the person is able to understand the information that is relevant to making [the] decision and able to appreciate the reasonably foreseeable consequences of [that] decision' (Bill 109 1992, p. 5). If a particular client is able to do this and has been declared incompetent, the therapist needs to urge reassessment and reinstatement of the client's basic civil rights.

Surrogate client centredness

There may be some occasions when a client is completely unable to express his or her wishes, such as a client in persistent vegetative state. There may be occasions when a client has been found legally incompetent and the decision to be made has significant risk or legal import. There may be occasions when a client is, in the therapist's opinion, medically incapable of making a reasoned decision for any one of a variety of reasons, including difficulty in understanding or remembering and utilizing relevant information and/or difficulty in appreciating the risks of a course of action. While it is an approach of last resort, in such circumstances, the occupational therapist should contact a surrogate decision-maker.

The identity of the appropriate surrogate may have been legally determined, particularly in cases where the individual has been found legally incompetent. In some jurisdictions,

---

Case study: Nick and the red wheelchair

'Nick' (a pseudonym) was a man in his early seventies who had sustained a left cerebral vascular accident. He had been left with right hemiplegia and some language difficulties, compounded by the fact that English was not Nick's first (or even second or third) language. He had learned English informally as a refugee in central Europe after World War II and on the job after immigration to Canada. He spoke English with a heavy accent.

Nick had no known family, and he lived in a long-term care hospital. He had had a neighbour managing his finances at one time, but his bank manager had initiated an investigation into misuse of his funds by this neighbour. Having been found legally incompetent to manage his financial affairs, and given the absence of a trustworthy friend or family member, his property was now under the control of a government-appointed trustee.

Nick needed a wheelchair. He could propel himself independently using his left arm and leg but, because he was unusually short, no chair available in the hospital was low enough to allow his feet to reach the floor comfortably. He would need to purchase his own super-low chair. Although a government funding programme would subsidise the purchase, Nick would need to expend personal funds to acquire the chair.

As his occupational therapist, the author discussed with Nick his need for a chair low enough for him to reach the floor comfortably. He immediately comprehended the idea of a 'new chair, just for me' and was eager to pursue it. Arrangements were made for several chairs to be brought in by a local vendor for trial.

As soon as Nick saw the assembled chairs, he stated that he wanted the 'red sports car', pointing to a wheelchair with a red frame and black upholstery. He indicated that this 'red sports car' would help him 'catch all the sexy girls'. The chair for which Nick expressed this preference was too wide. Other chairs fitted better, but he consistently stated that he wanted the 'red sports car'. When asked to consider elements of the chair other than colour, such as comfort, he would reiterate that he wanted the 'red sports car'.

Realising that this approach to wheelchair selection was too complex for Nick, several attempts were made to simplify the task. First, a sequence was imposed. The fit and comfort of the chair would be decided before addressing colour. Questions were phrased so as to eliminate the effect of colour, while addressing the priority characteristics. For example, Nick would be asked whether he would like this chair better than the red one if this one were also red. Under this circumstance, he responded in terms of the comfort of the chair or how easily he could 'drive' it. However, Nick still became overwhelmed by the array of choices, and he could not remember which chair was most comfortable.

The next modification to the decision-making process was to impose a framework. The number of options with which Nick had to deal at any one time was limited. Nick was assessed on only two chairs per appointment. Within this limited array, he was able to express clear and consistent messages about comfort and ease of propulsion, although the issue of colour arose at every session over the next several weeks.

Once the issues of fit, comfort and ease of propulsion were finalised, it was time to deal with the issue of colour. Nick had expressed a strong, sustained and consistent desire to have a red wheelchair. Before beginning to assess the various wheelchairs, funding and the fact that Nick would have to pay for the chair had been discussed. He was aware of the fact that he did not have control of his finances and indicated that they were controlled by 'the government'. When he was informed that there would be an additional cost to have a red chair and that this surcharge would not be subsidized by the government programme but would have to be entirely paid from his funds, Nick said: 'Is worth it.' He went on to say that he had 'never had sexy red sports car before' and that it would help him 'catch all the girls' now that he was no longer young. When he was reminded that the extra expenditure would have to be authorised by his trustee, he said: 'Is my money. I can pay.' It was time to implement advocacy.

A letter was sent to Nick's trustee clearly explaining the need for a wheelchair, the various necessary features, the total cost, the proportion subsidised and the outstanding expense against Nick's estate. No difficulty was anticipated in obtaining approval for this. The difficulty might arise over the extra cost of the colour option. The letter went on to explain the additional cost and the fact that this would not be subsidised. It also stated openly that this was not an entirely necessary expenditure. However, it went on to explain how sustained and consistent Nick's preference was, pointing out that he had even preferred a red chair over one he admitted was more comfortable. Nick's reason for wanting the red chair was not detailed, but the potential impact of colour on his acceptance of the wheelchair was mentioned. The letter also detailed Nick's awareness of both who managed his finances and the extra cost of the colour option and his belief it would be worth it and that he could afford it. The letter closed by urging the trustee to authorise the extra expense if Nick's finances allowed it.

individuals can appoint, while legally competent, a trusted person to act on their behalf should they become incompetent. Some jurisdictions have a legislated hierarchy, with the most senior person available taking responsibility (e.g. a spouse, if available, would be preferred to a child, who in turn would be preferred to a sibling). Should it become necessary to work with a surrogate, the occupational therapist will need to establish the identity of the appropriate individual.

This surrogate could then be consulted in lieu of the client, whenever client participation was needed but the client himself or herself could not make a particular reasoned decision. The therapist would play both educational and advocacy roles in this circumstance, ensuring that the surrogate recognised the responsibility to decide on the client's behalf, considering the client's previously expressed wishes or former values, habits and preferences rather than the surrogate decision-maker's own opinions.

CASE EXAMPLE

The case study of Nick and the red wheelchair is drawn from the author's clinical experience. It was this case that first sparked an interest in the topic of client-centred practice with clients with cognitive impairment. It is also where the strategies of graded decision-making and advocacy were first applied to this issue.

Some colleagues scoffed at the idea of advocating for a red chair for Nick. One stated that he probably would not even remember wanting a red one by the time his chair was delivered, and others derided the waste of time and effort, because the trustee would never approve such an unnecessary expenditure. As the occupational therapist in the case, this author never considered that this was a waste of time. Occupational therapists strive to be client centred, and these actions were directed to that end. Nick had participated in the decision-making process and had expressed a clear preference for a red chair. There was reason to believe that he was capable of making that decision, as demonstrated by the consistency of this desire over a period of several

weeks, his willingness to pay extra for this feature, and the fact that he had a clear rationale for his decision. The fact that he called the wheelchair a car or that others might not agree with his rationale was peripheral to the issue of capacity. He had passed the 'understand and appreciate test'.

In the end, the trustee assented and Nick got his red chair. That decision provided some degree of vindication in the eyes of colleagues, but the use of a client-centred approach, adapted by graded decision-making and advocacy, was appropriate whatever the outcome. There is support for this stand in an informal poll of approximately 60 occupational therapists working with clients with cognitive impairment. They enthusiastically agreed that occupational therapists should listen to and respect clients' opinions and preferences, even when the client has cognitive impairments and/or has been found legally incompetent (Hobson 1996).

CONCLUSION

Occupational therapists treat many clients with cognitive impairments, and these clients are particularly vulnerable to having their capacity to participate in client-centred care questioned. Although this style of care does make significant cognitive demands of clients, the therapist still can and should practise client-centred occupational therapy with individuals with cognitive impairment. To that end, this chapter has outlined four strategies to assist the therapist:

- *Enhanced client assessment* will allow an occupational therapist to learn as much as possible about the client and understand his or her decision-making abilities. Every occupational therapist engages in *clinical capacity assessment* to determine whether each client is medically capable of making reasoned decisions about care. This may extend to more formal assessment of cognitive abilities or even assessment of legal competence in some cases. During *extended history-taking*, the therapist consults individuals who know the client well to help understand the client's habits, preferences and style of communicating.

- *Graded decision-making* is a method of adapting the activity of decision-making to accommodate the client's cognitive impairments. The therapist assists the client in making appropriate decisions, delicately balancing some degree of client-centred practice, including elements such as choice and autonomy, with an appropriate professional concern for client safety. The therapist may want to consider the inherent risks associated with individual decisions and foster more choice and autonomy when the risk is low.
- *Advocacy* on behalf of a client is not new to occupational therapists, but it is particularly important when the client has cognitive impairment. Such clients are often presumed incapable of having any input into decisions about their care, whereas even clients found legally incompetent may be able to express their wishes. The occupational therapist can advocate for these with team members and others responsible for the care of these clients.
- As a last resort, the occupational therapist may need to practise a form of *surrogate client-centredness*, where a surrogate decision-maker is consulted in lieu of the client himself or herself. Advocacy is closely linked with this form of practice, to ensure that the surrogate understands that he or she is acting in the client's stead.

With these adaptations, it is possible to practise client-centred occupational therapy with persons with cognitive impairment, but that is not to say that it is easy. In fact, this may be the true test of an occupational therapist's skill and will. Such practice combines the art and science of occupational therapy. The science is revealed in particularly skilled assessment and activity adaptation. The art lies in establishing the degree of trust and rapport needed to allow the therapist to understand and interpret the wishes of these clients to others guiding their care. Deciding to practise client-centred care with persons with cognitive impairment also constitutes a test of will, because it is so easy, and acceptable, to justify non-client-centred care with this population. Colleagues may decry your actions as noble but unrealistic. Some genuinely believe that it is impossible, whereas others may be guiltily aware that you are attempting something they have not.

Despite the fact that client-centred care with persons with cognitive impairment can form the ultimate test of a therapist's commitment to this style of practice, occupational therapists are invited to rise to the challenge. Others have tried and succeeded, and clients deserve therapists' every effort. One recent study of client-centred care from the perspective of individuals with experience of mental illness and the mental health-care system sums the reason in its title: 'Client-centred care means I am a valued human being' (Corring 1996). If occupational therapists believe that their clients are 'valued human beings' and wish to demonstrate that in their interactions with them, therapists must offer them client-centred care, whatever the impairments that led them to seek occupational therapy services.

REFERENCES

Alzheimer's Disease Society 1998
http://www.vois.org.uk/alzheimers
Anderson J M, Waxler-Morrison N, Richardson N, Herbert C, Murphy M 1990 Conclusion: delivering culturally sensitive health care. In: Waxler-Morrison N, Anderson J, Richardson E (eds) Cross-cultural caring: a handbook for health professionals. University of British Columbia Press, Vancouver, ch 10, pp 245–267
Appelbaum P S, Grisso T 1988 Assessing patients' capacities to consent to treatment. New England Journal of Medicine 319(25):1635–1638

Bill 109 1992 An act respecting consent to treatment, 1992 Statutes of Ontario. Queen's Printer for Ontario, Toronto
Canadian Association of Occupational Therapists 1991 Occupational therapy guidelines for client-centred practice. Canadian Association of Occupational Therapists, Toronto
Canadian Study of Health and Aging Working Group 1994 Canadian study of health and aging: study methods and prevalence of dementia. Canadian Medical Association Journal 150(6):899–912

Corring D J 1996 Client-centred care means I am a valued human being. Master's thesis, The University of Western Ontario, London

Curtin L L 1995 Good intentions pave the road … Nursing Management 26(2):7–8

Dihn D, Ganesan S, Waxler-Morrison N 1990 The Vietnamese. In: Waxler-Morrison N, Anderson J, Richardson E (eds) Cross-cultural caring: a handbook for health professionals. University of British Columbia Press, Vancouver, ch 8, pp 181–213

Fiesta J 1992 Refusal of treatment. Nursing Management 23(11):14–18

Fleming M H 1991 The therapist with the three-track mind. American Journal of Occupational Therapy 45(11):1007–1014

Fulbrook P 1994 Assessing mental competence of patients and relatives. Journal of Advanced Nursing 20:457–461

Gage M, Polatajko H 1995 Naming practice: the case for the term client-driven. Canadian Journal of Occupational Therapy 62(3):115–118

Giles G M, Clark-Wilson J 1993 Brain injury rehabilitation: a neurofacilitatory approach. Chapman & Hall, London

Hobson S J G 1996 Being client-centred when the client is cognitively impaired. Canadian Journal of Occupational Therapy 63(2):133–137

Lai M C, Yue K K 1990 The Chinese. In: Waxler-Morrison N, Anderson J, Richardson E (eds) Cross-cultural caring: a handbook for health professionals. University of British Columbia Press, Vancouver, ch 4, pp 68–90

Law M, Baptiste S, Carswell-Opzoomer A, McColl M A, Polatajko H, Pollock N 1991 Canadian Occupational Performance Measure. Canadian Association of Occupational Therapists, Toronto

Law M, Baptiste S, Mills J 1995 Client-centred practice: what does it mean and does it make a difference? Canadian Journal of Occupational Therapy 62(5):250–257

National Schizophrenia Fellowship 1998 http://www.nsf.org.uk

Okabe T, Takahashi K, Richardson E 1990 The Japanese. In: Waxler-Morrison N, Anderson J, Richardson E (eds) Cross-cultural caring: a handbook for health professionals. University of British Columbia Press, Vancouver, ch 6, pp 116–140

Ontario Ministry of the Attorney General 1996a Regulation no. 243/96. Queen's Printer for Ontario, Toronto

Ontario Ministry of the Attorney General 1996b Form C: assessment form. Queen's Printer for Ontario, Toronto

Ontario Ministry of Health 1994 Consent to treatment: a guide to the Act. Queens Printer for Ontario, Toronto

Richardson E 1990 The Cambodians and Laotians. In: Waxler-Morrison N, Anderson J, Richardson E (eds) Cross-cultural caring: a handbook for health professionals. University of British Columbia Press, Vancouver, ch 2, pp 11–35

Rogers C R 1951 Client-centred therapy: its current practice, implications, and theory. Houghton Mifflin, Boston

Silberfeld M 1992 New directions in assessing mental competence. Canadian Family Physician 38:2365–2369

Statistics Canada 1986 Report on the Canadian health and disability survey 1983–1984. Supply and Services Canada, Ottawa

Statistics Canada 1994 Selected characteristics of persons with disabilities residing in households: 1991 health and activity limitations survey. Statistics Canada, Ottawa

Sumsion T 1993 Client-centred practice: the true impact. Canadian Journal of Occupational Therapy 60(1):6–8

Thomas C L (ed) 1997 Taber's cyclopedic medical dictionary. F A Davis, Philadelphia

Toomey M, Nicholson D, Carswell A 1995 The clinical utility of the Canadian Occupational Performance Measure. Canadian Journal of Occupational Therapy 62(5):242–249

Venesy B A 1994 A clinician's guide to decision making capacity and ethically sound medical decisions. American Journal of Physical Medicine and Rehabilitation 73(3):219–226

Waters D 1995 Recovering from a depressive episode using the Canadian Occupational Performance Measure. Canadian Journal of Occupational Therapy 62(5):278–282

Yerxa E J, Clark F, Frank G et al 1989 An introduction to occupational science, a foundation for occupational therapy in the 21st century. Occupational Therapy in Health Care 6(4):1–17

Zoltan B 1990 Evaluation and treatment of cognitive dysfunction. In: Pedretti LW, Zoltan B (eds) Occupational therapy: practice skills for physical dysfunction. Mosby, St Louis, ch 12, pp 202–209

7

Using a client-centred approach with elderly people

S. J. G. Hobson

Demographic changes mean that occupational therapists will be treating ever more older adults. Unique characteristics of this population that present potential barriers to client-centred care, including health status and attitudes, are discussed. Specific recommendations are made for facilitating a client-centred approach with older adults.

The world is experiencing what has been termed an 'age wave' (Dychtwald & Flower 1990), and this is even more pronounced in the more developed countries (Office of Gerontological Studies 1996). Dychtwald & Flower (1990) identify three factors contributing to this shift in demographics. Longevity has increased for older adults, particularly in the more developed countries, where medical advances have extended life expectancy. Another factor is the declining birth rate. A third factor, which is accelerating the effect of the other two, particularly in North America, is the ageing of the post-World War II 'baby boom'. The eldest members of this cohort turn 65 in the year 2011.

Overall, the fastest growing segment of the population is those over the age of 65 years and, of those, the old-old (individuals aged over 85 years) are the fastest growing sector (Dychtwald & Flower 1990). In 1994, the elderly constituted 18.2% of the population in the UK, or some ten million people (Age Concern England 1997). The expected growth rate for those aged over 65 years is only 2% over the next 10 years, but this is no cause for complacency. The number of individuals over the age of 75 is expected to double over the next 50 years, while the number of those aged over 90 is expected to increase five-fold (Age Concern England 1997). In Canada, the proportion of the population aged over 65 years is lower, but faster growing, with 11.6% over the age of 65 in 1991 (Office of Gerontological Studies 1996), or some 3.2 million individuals (National Advisory Council on Aging (NACA) 1993a). This proportion is expected to double by the year 2031, but once again the oldest group, those aged over 85 years, will grow faster, almost tripling (Office of Gerontological Studies 1996).

Given these numbers, it should have become clear why a separate chapter has been allocated for the discussion of client-centred care with elderly people. Most occupational therapists will have some exposure to the care of those aged over 65, and for many therapists this group will form the majority of clients seen.

This chapter starts with a brief description of the population under discussion. The focus is then turned to barriers to various elements of client-centred care experienced by older clients. It should be understood that some younger clients may face similar barriers and that not all older adults will experience them to the same extent. None the less, the barriers discussed are more prevalent among elderly clients. The barriers faced relate to the typical life circumstances of the elderly, their health status, and the attitudes of both the elderly clients themselves and health-care professionals. Strategies to help overcome these barriers and foster client-centred care will be identified.

The constituent elements of client-centred care that will be considered in this chapter have been drawn from two sources. Law et al (1997) define client-centred practice as demonstrating respect for clients, involving clients in decision-making, advocating with and for clients, and recognising clients' experience and knowledge. A slightly different list of elements from Law and co-workers (1995) includes autonomy and choice, partnership and responsibility, enablement, contextual congruence, accessibility and flexibility, and respect for diversity. All of these elements will be considered in this chapter.

PIONEERS IN AGEING

Given that few have lived to what we now consider old age until very recently, today's elderly have been described as pioneers (Kiernat 1991). Occupational therapists seeking to offer client-centred care to older adults first need to understand their environments and culture so that therapy can be contextually congruent (Law et al 1995). Individual older clients may be more or less typical of their cohort, but it is useful to understand the cohort realities in order to view the client holistically, frame appropriate assessment questions, and recognise how unique a given client's experience may be. This section will consider some of the life circumstances typical of the cohort now pioneering old age that occupational therapists routinely consider when planning treatment, such as living arrangements and the availability of financial resources (see Table 7.1).

Women live longer than men, so the older client is more apt to be a woman, and she is apt to be a widow. Should the client be a man, he is probably still married, and thus may be expected to have more social support available (Age Concern England 1997, Office of Gerontological Studies 1996; see also Table 7.1). The older client will probably live in his or her own home (see Table 7.1), but as age advances so does the probability of moving into rented accommodation or of being placed in an institution (Office of Gerontological Studies 1996). Canadian rates of institutionalization are higher than those in England (Forbes et al 1987; see also Table 7.1). Factors such as population mobility, climate, geography, and the number of women in the workforce have been suggested as contributing to this (Schwenger & Gross 1980).

Both the UK and Canada have government-sponsored income support programmes, and many older adults rely heavily upon these. In 51% of pensioner households in the UK at least 75% of income is from state pensions and benefits (Age Concern England 1997), and 60% of income for single Canadians aged over 65 years comes from government programmes (NACA 1996). Such supports are not generous, however, and most older adults have less discretionary

Table 7.1 Life circumstances of the population aged over 65 years in the UK and Canada

Attribute	UK	Canada
Gender distribution		
65+	1.5 women per man*	1.4 women per man
85+	3 women per man*	2.3 women per man
Marital status		
65+	75% of men married†	77% of men married
	51% of women married†	43% of women married
75+	60% of men married†	73% of men married
	23% of women married†	30% of women married
Housing		
65+	55% own, no mortgage†	60% own, no mortgage
	9% own, mortgage†	6% own, mortgage
	36% rent†	27% rent
Institutionalisation		
65–74	1.0%‡	1.9% of men
		2.0% of women
75–84	5.5%‡	7.0% of men
		10.4% of women
85+	25.2%‡	25.5% of men
		38.8% of women
Affluence	Senior households spend 1/11 more of their income on food and shelter than other households (41.5% vs 38.2%)	Senior households spend 1/7 more of their income on food and shelter than other households (38.9% vs 33.9%)

* UK; † Great Britain; ‡ England.
Sources: Age Concern England 1997, Office of Gerontological Studies 1996.

income than younger adults (see Table 7.1). This is worth considering, because 'adequate income is critical to the health, well-being, and standard of living of older people' (NACA 1991, p. 1). The financial ability of older adults to participate in leisure occupations, something of interest to occupational therapists, may be especially compromised.

Canada and the UK both have socialised medicine, whereby basic medical care is provided free at the point of need to all citizens. However, in some jurisdictions, some health-related expenses (e.g. medications, assistive devices, etc.) are not fully covered. Britain has broader health-care coverage than Canada (Novak 1993), particularly in terms of the development of community health-care initiatives, which were not funded under Canada's early Medicare system (NACA 1995). This lack of home health-care funding has been implicated in the higher rate of institutionalization in Canada (Schwenger & Gross 1980). The UK has 'official guidelines [that] call for 1.5 full time equivalent home help aides per thousand population ... compared to an estimate in the early 1980s of 0.5 per thousand in Canada' (Forbes et al 1987, p. 49). This sector of health care has grown rapidly in Canada, and the number of home support workers and agencies for seniors 'increased by at least 50% in the last decade' (NACA 1993c). Use of formal supports is linked to increasing disability and to lower levels of informal assistance (Stone & DeWit 1991). It is important to note, however, that it is not a case of using either formal or informal supports. Often both are needed. Informal caregivers may access formal supports when the strain of caring undermines their own health or to supplement their informal care efforts (NACA 1995).

Beyond considering the formal supports available to the elderly, it is equally or more important to consider informal supports, because 'friends and family members provide between 75% and 85% of the help received by seniors needing care in the community' (NACA 1993c). Such informal support is three times as likely to come from women as men, and spouses and daughters are the primary caregivers (NACA 1990). Male and female carers tend to approach informal care differently, performing different types of tasks and offering different types of support (NACA 1990, Turk-Charles et al 1996). Women usually provide direct personal care and offer emotional support, whereas men typically assist with financial matters and home maintenance and offer instrumental support, such as managing care. Particularly where the primary carer is the spouse, it is important to recognise that the caregiver may be just as elderly as the client. In Great Britain, of those devoting at least 20 hours per week to caring, 28% were aged over 65 years (Age Concern England 1997). Even when the caregiver is an adult child, the carer may also be elderly. As many as 25% of those aged between 65 and 74 and 10% of those aged over 75 have a living parent who may require care at some future date (Stone et al 1987).

BARRIERS TO CLIENT-CENTRED CARE AND STRATEGIES TO OVERCOME THESE

Some basic cohort differences between the elderly and other adults in the general population have been discussed; however, there are many other differences between these two groups that relate specifically to the context of health care. Two main categories of differences between younger and older adult as clients will be discussed in this chapter. These are the overall health status of the clients and the attitudes held by the clients and many health-care workers. Both present potential barriers to client-centred care.

Health status

There is a widespread perception that older adulthood is characterized by ill health and dependency. This is only partially true. Disability rises with age, as does prescription drug use (Office of Gerontological Studies 1996) and average length of hospital stay (Age Concern England 1997). However, this gives a distorted image.

'Most older people do not need or use excessive amounts of health care' (Novak 1993, p. 203), and only 20% of Canadian seniors report that they require assistance in daily living (NACA 1993b). A longitudinal study in the province of Manitoba, Canada, showed that less than one-quarter of seniors had a hospital stay in any given year, and almost three-fifths of the hospital days were used by only 5% of the older population (Roos et al 1984). Further, the older population made only 1.7 more visits to their physicians per year than those aged 15–44 years, and only 0.9 more visits per year than those aged 45–64 (Roos et al 1984). In fact, 74% of Canadian seniors rate their health as good, very good or excellent (Office of Gerontological Studies 1996)

In this section, several specific topics related to health status will be discussed in more detail, identifying what barriers they may present to client-centred care. These include sensory change, co-morbidity and frailty, and environmental vulnerability. Specific recommendation about how to implement client-centred care in the face of these barriers will follow each subsection.

Sensory change

The acuity of all sensory systems declines with age, although not all senses decline at the same rate (Levy 1986). Taste, touch, smell and vestibular senses, while all affected and important, will not be the focus here, as changes in these have less direct impact on client-centred care than changes in vision and hearing.

Hearing loss associated with the ageing process, known as presbycusis, is conservatively estimated to affect over 50% of those aged over 60 years (Lai 1990). This form of loss is not necessarily a complete inability to hear; it is more often associated with difficulty in discriminating sounds, particularly speech (Lai 1990). As such, it leads to enormous frustration and anxiety in social situations, and it certainly presents a barrier to a client-centred relationship.

There are many causes of visual deterioration in later life. These include presbyopia (the poor accommodation for close vision associated with ageing), cataracts, glaucoma and diabetic retinopathy (Naeyaert 1990). The leading cause of visual deterioration in later life, however, is macular degeneration, where the centre of the individual's field of vision deteriorates and vision in this field becomes blurred. Macular degeneration alone accounts for 45% of new visual losses reported annually (Naeyaert 1990). Overall, approximately 1 in 10 of those over the age of 65 has a visual loss significant enough to interfere with daily living (Naeyaert 1990). Again, such deficits will naturally impact on the care of affected clients.

Client-centred strategy: enhanced communication

Care cannot be client centred without effective communication between client and therapist. Clients needs to be able to receive and comprehend information and express their autonomous choices at every stage of the process, from assessment through to outcome measurement. Given the marked hearing and/or visual losses of so many older adults (Lai 1990, Naeyaert 1990), therapists must be careful to assure optimal communication so that clients can participate in the decision-making process, as mandated in client-centred care (Law et al 1995, 1997). Selecting therapeutic settings with low ambient noise and high ambient lighting (but no glare) is sometimes a challenge in busy departments or the client's hectic home, but such efforts will optimise communication with all clients, especially older ones.

There are many resources available that suggest ways to accommodate for the hearing loss (see Orange & Ryan 1995) and visual decline (see Cooper 1985, Kolanowski 1992) associated with the ageing process. However, most fail to mention such basic strategies as ensuring that clients are wearing the glasses and/or hearing-aids that they require and that these are functional. It seems hard to image that this could be overlooked, but many therapists do not seem to know how to turn on hearing-aids, check that the batteries are charged, or adjust the volume. Clients have also said: 'You're the only one who ever washes my glasses.'

Ensuring that assessment materials and home programmes are available in larger font is important for clients with visual impairment. It is also vital to consider the reading level required in all written home programmes and client educational material. One-third of older adults have only elementary education, with this proportion rising with age (Office of Gerontological Studies 1996). A client who cannot hear, see or read therapeutic information cannot effectively participate in the therapeutic partnership. Further, failure to assure these basics implies a lack of respect for the client, which is another element central to client-centred care (Law et al 1997).

Co-morbidity and frailty

A co-morbid disease is one that coexists with the primary reason for seeking health care. The elderly are more likely to display co-morbidity than younger adult clients, primarily because of their likelihood of having chronic health problems. These chronic health conditions include, in descending frequency, arthritis, hypertension and respiratory problems (Office of Gerontological Studies 1996). In Canada, 80% of those aged over 65 years reported one or more chronic conditions (NACA 1993b), whereas in Great Britain only 63% of those over the age of 75 reported a long-standing health problem (Age Concern England 1997). Recognising the presence of co-morbid conditions is essential to good health care, as these conditions may complicate and/or prolong recovery from the presenting diagnosis. For example, a client admitted for a hip fracture may find recovery complicated by the presence of arthritis in the knees and hands, which could impede use of assistive devices, such as a walking frame.

A concomitant of having multiple health problems is an increased probability of taking multiple prescription (Office of Gerontological Studies 1996) and over-the-counter medications (Yee & Williams 1996). This polypharmacy may complicate an older client's recovery because of the increased risk of toxic interactions among medications. All health-care professionals involved with the older client must be alert to this possibility, but occupational therapists, who often visit the client's home, may be in the best position to discover the extent of polypharmacy.

Because many older adults already have one or more chronic health problems (Age Concern England 1997, NACA 1993b), they are often labelled 'frail', meaning that they are vulnerable to other health problems. These include secondary medical complications (Brummel-Smith 1990), medication misuse (Yee & Williams 1996) and malnourishment (Chernoff 1996). Further, the ill-effects of these problems are greater in older clients. Brummel-Smith (1990) suggests that once one thing extra goes wrong, the elderly client can suffer a 'cascade of disasters' (p. 7), wherein an escalating series of adverse reactions can have disastrous results. He gives the example of a patient who starts with a simple respiratory infection, has an adverse reaction to antihistamine medication, falls, and thereafter proceeds to experience immobility and a variety of complications that ultimately end with the individual being placed in a care facility or even dying. While this seems an extreme example, for older adults who are having difficulty coping, even a minor ailment may push them across the threshold to being non-functional and/or requiring formal health supports. With their emphasis on self-care occupations, including managing one's own health, occupational therapists have a role to play in minimising the health risks of frailty.

The problems of co-morbidity and frailty threaten client-centred practice in several ways. First, they influence the attitude of both the client and the health-care professional. They reinforce negative stereotypes about ageing and foster an attitude of what could be called therapeutic nihilism, a belief that therapeutic intervention would be useless. These will be addressed in greater detail later in the chapter, under the headings of ageism and health beliefs, along with strategies to counter them.

In addition, co-morbidity and frailty contribute to the extremely complex nature of the health-care problems of the elderly. Because of this complexity, the interdisciplinary health-care team has been described as the 'basic unit of geriatric care' (Zeiss & Steffen 1996, p. 423).

Multiple practitioners each focus on the presenting problems that lie within their specific scope of practice. Naturally, this type of professional specialisation can lead to fragmented care. While teams working in geriatrics are urged to obtain patient input, or at least reaction (Brummel-Smith 1990), this does not go as far as client-centred practice demands. Further, even this limited client consultation does not always happen.

Client-centred strategy: advocacy

Advocacy with and for clients is part of client-centred occupational therapy (Law et al 1997). An important role for a client-centred therapist is as an advocate for full participation by the older client as a member of the team, whenever possible. When this is not possible, for whatever reason, the therapist should at least ensure that the client's voice is heard by the team. Further, health-care teams often operate in the medical model, with an emphasis on the problem and/or diagnosis. This can compound the fragmentation of care mentioned above. It is the responsibility of a client-centred therapist to consider the client as an individual who is more than the sum of his or her various health-care problems and to present this holistic image of the client to the team. This is part of respecting the client. Reductionism is incongruent with client-centred practice.

Environmental vulnerability

It is certainly understandable that, because of the sensory changes related to ageing, older adults are at greater risk than younger ones of misinterpreting environmental cues. Visual decline, in fact, is considered a major cause of falls in older adults (Tobias et al 1990). However, the concept that will be introduced here goes beyond this simple understanding of environmental vulnerability to the work of Lawton.

The model of competency–press suggests that behaviour is related to the interaction of the individual's competencies and the press within the environment (Lawton & Nahemow 1973). Competencies refer to the individual's cognitive ability, psychological adjustment and physical health; press refers to the degree of demand within the environment as perceived by the individual. The model postulates that a balance between press and competency is necessary for positive affect and adaptive behaviour. It also postulates that environmental demands that are incongruent with the individual's competency, either greater or lesser, lead to negative affect and maladaptive behaviour (Lawton & Nahemow 1973).

The competency–press model is widely discussed in gerontological literature because of an associated hypothesis. The environmental docility hypothesis proposes that as the competence of the individual decreases the influence of environment on the individual's behaviour increases (Lawton & Nahemow 1973). This hypothesis suggests increased environmental vulnerability for the elderly, whose competencies may be diminishing. Lawton (1985) later supplemented this somewhat negative hypothesis with the environmental proactivity hypothesis, which states that individuals with higher levels of competence will better use the resources within the environment.

The environmental docility hypothesis (Lawton & Nahemow 1973) offers one explanation for the greater difficulty that older adults have in adjusting to new surroundings, such as the confusion often seen initially after admission to hospital, or the relatively greater stress demonstrated in response to the advent of a home health worker into the client's home. It is also interesting to note that both of these hypotheses are congruent with occupational therapy theory and practice, wherein the environment is seen both as an intrinsic factor in the client's occupational performance and a legitimate avenue of intervention.

Client-centred strategy: client control

Perhaps the hallmark of client-centred practice is to allow the client choice and control throughout the therapeutic process. This truly allows the client to participate meaningfully in decision-making. This is exactly what is mandated by the competency–press model.

At one level, the client needs choice about the level of environmental stimulation and resources. The more competent client needs to exercise choice in utilizing environmental resources, while the less competent client needs choice so that excess stimulation in the environment can be eliminated. The client-centred therapist must involve the older client in decisions about levels of environmental stimulation and support.

On a more fundamental level, however, occupational therapists must recognise the responsibility placed upon the client in the client-centred practice model. This creates a high level of environmental press. Although this may be ideal for more competent clients, less competent clients may find the press excessive, which could lead to negative affect and maladaptive behaviour. The client-centred therapist must be prepared to moderate the demands for decision-making placed on the less competent elderly client in order to ensure optimum press. By adjusting the level of client control in response to the client's needs, the therapist is being truly client centred.

Attitudes

Perhaps more than health status, some of the attitudes of the elderly influence client-centred practice. Attitudes have a pervasive and subtle influence on all behaviours, so attitudes toward the ageing process and about the elderly will affect health-care delivery when working with older adults. People learn attitudes from significant others and from life experiences (Shilton 1995), so naturally attitudes vary among cultures (Bonder 1994). The roles of the media and of humour in attitude development have also been recognised (Novak 1993). This section will consider some of the attitudinal influences unique to working with the elderly, including ageism, health beliefs, patterns of under-reporting health problems, and the potential influence of the life experiences of older clients, that may create barriers to a client-centred approach. Again, specific strategies to facilitate client-centred care will be discussed after each subsection.

Ageism

Ageism is a form of prejudice, literally prejudge-ment, linked to age; it usually refers to negative stereotypes about old age. Ageist attitudes are common in Western culture, and the term 'geron-tophobia' has even been reported in the literature (Helm 1987). Neither individual health-care pro-fessionals nor the health-care system are immune from ageism, and this is demonstrated in reluc-tance to work in the field of geriatrics, setting lower goals for older clients (Kiernat 1991, Shilton 1995) or selectively remembering the clients' deficits more clearly than their strengths (Edelstein & Semenchuk 1996). It is clear then that ageism presents a threat to accessibility, an element of client-centred care identified by Law et al (1995). Fortunately, there is evidence to sug-gest that occupational therapy students' attitudes toward the elderly are somewhat more positive, possibly because of relatively high knowledge levels (Todd et al 1986).

It is also important to remember that elderly clients themselves may hold ageist attitudes, including 'beliefs that persons their age cannot recover or adapt to a disability' (Brummel-Smith 1990, p. 16). These attitudes may be reinforced by their health status, if they are frail or experience multiple health problems. Another source of reinforcement for these negative feelings may be the way they are treated, based on their physical appearance and the stereotypes of ageing that it may provoke. Orange and Ryan (1995) describe a 'communication predicament' (p. 121) faced by older adults when those around them act on stereotyped expectations about the elderly and modify their communication patterns (e.g. speaking more loudly, simplifying messages and posing closed questions). These altered commu-nication patterns constrain the communication opportunities available to the older person and elicit stereotyped response behaviours (e.g. single-word replies), resulting in loss of self-esteem and reduced social interaction for the older adult. In this scenario, both the older person and those interacting with him or her have negative stereotypes and attitudes reinforced, establishing a vicious cycle of ageism.

Client-centred strategies: advocacy, therapeutic use of self, and enhanced communication

The health-care environment is not immune to ageism. This may be demonstrated overtly, when clients are labelled 'bed-blockers' to imply that they somehow have less right to occupy a hospi-tal bed than younger patients, or more subtly, when older clients receive less direct treatment time (Shilton 1995). One of the elements of client-centred practice is ensuring that the client has access to services (Law et al 1995), and this may require the therapist to challenge ageist attitudes in colleagues or within the health-care system itself to ensure that older clients have equitable access to care. Advocating with and for the client is an element of client-centred practice (Law et al 1995) that becomes even more impor-tant in helping to ensure that older clients receive the treatment they need.

In recent years, attention has focused on the client's contribution to the therapeutic relation-ship, and the phrase 'therapeutic use of self', with its emphasis on the therapist's actions and attitudes, has fallen into disuse. However, the therapist still has tremendous influence within the therapeutic relationship, and there are times when it is appropriate to exercise this.

Occupational therapists cannot practise client-centred care based on ageist attitudes, given that respect for clients is one of the elements of the client-centred approach (Law et al 1997), as is the positive, ability-focused, enablement approach (Law et al 1995). Although some authors urge optimism (Kiernat 1991) or enthusiasm (Helm 1987) when treating older adults, probably as an antidote to systemic ageism, the more appropri-ate route is to examine personal attitudes to treating older people to be sure that these are not adversely influencing treatment decisions (Brummel-Smith 1990, Helm 1987), to challenge overt instances of therapeutic hopelessness (Brummel-Smith 1990), and to work towards set-ting goals that are realistic (Andrews 1987, Davis 1996) for every client, regardless of age. The therapist's conscious use of self to demonstrate genuine respect for the older client can help restore client self-esteem. Over-optimism or hearty encouragement are really forms of conde-scension, and such therapeutic dishonesty will undermine the partnership between client and therapist that is a defining characteristic of client-centred care.

Another strategy important in combating ageist attitudes and promoting client-centred care is enhanced communication. This was addressed earlier in the chapter in a simpler form, accommodating sensory changes; how-ever, those suggestions did not address the attitudinal barriers to effective communication outlined above in the communication predica-ment model. To break the vicious cycle described there, Orange and Ryan (1995) propose a 'communication enhancement model' (p. 129). Within this model, individuals encountering an older person consider the potential communi-cation adjustments that may be needed but do not implement these until they have tested whether the adjustments are actually necessary. Modifying communication only as needed empowers both parties and leads to effective communication (Orange & Ryan 1995). Use of the communication enhancement model will demonstrate respect for the client, optimise com-munication, and foster the partnership between client and therapist sought in client-centred care.

Health beliefs

Individuals have widely varying conceptions about what health is (van Maanen 1988), as well as about what causes illness and, therefore, what treatments are most likely to be effective (Waxler-Morrison 1990). Health and illness beliefs are strongly influenced by culture (Waxler-Morrison 1990) and sociodemographic factors such as gender, age, education, income and social connections (Galanos et al 1994, Strain 1989). Two aspects of health beliefs will be discussed here: attitudes towards health professionals and self-efficacy.

Older adults perceive the medical professions more positively and rate their medical care more highly than younger adults (Thorson & Powell 1991). Such attitudes about health professionals may lead older clients to assume a passive role in health-care interactions, either because they revere the professional (Thorson & Powell 1991) or because they are intimidated by his or her knowledge (Hofland 1992). Extreme regard for health professionals may lead the older client to fear taking too much of the professional's time or unrealistically to expect the professional to know what is wrong without needing to be told (Hofland 1992). This may lead to underreporting health concerns, which will be discussed next. Attitudes of exaggerated regard or intimidation are equally undesirable in terms of establishing the partnership mandated by client-centred care, because the passive role they inspire contradicts the premise of client involvement in treatment planning.

Another important consideration under the general heading of health beliefs is self-efficacy. Self-efficacy is closely allied to the concept of internal causation described in Kielhofner's (1985) model of human occupation; both refer to the individual's anticipation of success or mas-tery. Self-efficacy affects both initiation and per-sistence of coping efforts (Bandura 1978) and mediates anxiety responses (Bandura & Adams 1977). Self-efficacy with regard to health status is the extent to which people believe that they can influence their own health. This health belief has a potentially huge impact on client-centred health practice, given that its founding principle was that clients retain responsibility (Rogers 1951) for resolving their problems.

Waller and Bates (1992), in their study of healthy elderly, found that those with high self-efficacy believed that they were in control of their health and were more likely to engage in good health practices; however, Thorson and Powell (1991) reported that younger adults are more likely than older adults to hold a belief in taking responsibility for their own health. Self-efficacy may be a contributing factor to this finding.

Bandura (1978) identified four sources of self-efficacy information: performance levels, vicari-ous experience, verbal persuasion and aversive arousal (the unpleasant physiological symptoms of negative emotions, particularly anxiety). Abler and Fretz (1988) have suggested that all of these may be negatively affected for older adults, leaving them at greater risk of experiencing low self-efficacy. The ageing process may adversely affect individuals' performance and thus reduce self-efficacy. The vicarious experience obtained by seeing peers in ill health may have a negative impact on older adults' health self-efficacy. The ageism pervasive in Western culture may lower self-efficacy by means of verbal persuasion. Lastly, older adults may experience an increased physiological response to anxiety, also lowering self-efficacy (Abler & Fretz 1988). Low self-efficacy is a barrier to client-centred therapy, in that self-efficacy is linked to anticipation of success. Clients who do not believe that they can positively affect their health status will not be as likely to take an active role in therapy. Client passivity is antithetical to client-centred care.

Client-centred strategies: education, client control and promoting self-efficacy

Because of their respect for medical professionals (Thorson & Powell 1991), some older adults may prefer to rely on the professional's advice and feel very uncomfortable with the idea of telling the professional how therapy ought to proceed. Therapists seeking to establish a client-centred relationship with a client need to assess the client's attitude toward health professionals. The client will need to be told what client-centred care entails, highlighting the roles and responsibilities of each partner in the relationship. Exaggerated respect for or awe of professionals will need gentle redirection to include an awareness of the unique knowledge and contribution that the client brings to the partnership. Once the client understands his or her role, and as the professional demonstrates genuine respect for the client's knowledge and invites increasing contributions, the client may begin to participate more readily.

Until the client is comfortable with the responsibilities inherent in client-centred care, the therapist may need to be open to allowing the client to limit the degree of client control, hoping to increase client participation and progress to a true partnership. If older adults do not believe in taking responsibility for their own health as much as younger ones (Thorson & Powell 1991), this may be reflected in taking less responsibility for therapy decisions. One strategy for encouraging clients to exercise more control that this author has found successful is to provide the information needed for informed decision-making, explain why the information is germane, and offer advice only after the client has had the opportunity to consider this information. This process makes the therapeutic rationale clear and offers the client the opportunity to form an opinion and compare it with the therapist's advice. Each time this process is used it offers the client the opportunity to express an opinion should he or she so wish. Some clients have voiced their opinion at decision points later in the therapeutic relationship, presumably having gained confidence in their ability to formulate sound therapeutic decisions. Another strategy that works well for some decisions (e.g. selection of therapeutic activities) is to offer a range of choices with similar benefits and explain this similarity. This reduces the risk that a client may perceive in making a therapeutic decision.

Another method that may be used to foster client participation in therapy is to try to enhance self-efficacy directly, thereby giving clients a sense of control over their health. 'Nothing succeeds like success' is an old maxim with application to the concept of self-efficacy. Actual performance is considered the most influential source of self-efficacy information (Bandura 1978), so enabling performance will foster increased self-efficacy and, thus, may result in greater involvement in both therapy and the client-centred partnership. Careful selection of achievable goals and subsequent success may stimulate an upward spiral of self-efficacy and active participation in the client-centred process of care. A second method of enhancing self-efficacy is vicarious experience. Occupational therapists seeking to enhance client participation can use peer support to foster increased self-efficacy. While only 3% of those aged over 65 report being involved in self-help groups (Minister of National Health and Welfare 1993), 'the help given to seniors requiring assistance is often provided by another senior, most often the spouse, or by age peers' (Angus 1991,

p. 11). Linking your elderly clients with other older adults who have succeeded at therapy may prove beneficial by providing positive vicarious experiences that will enhance self-efficacy. It is also worth noting that the education process used to teach a client about client-centred care may act as a form of verbal persuasion. As the therapist explains the importance of client participation in the process, clients may come to believe in their influence over their own health.

Underreporting

Both ageism and health beliefs are closely tied to the problem of underreporting of health concerns, a significant issue among the elderly. Particularly prone to be underreported are pain (Hofland 1992), incontinence (Hood 1987), falls (Tideiksaar 1994) and elder abuse (McDonald et al 1995). One of the commonest reasons for failing to report health problems is fear of loss of control when the health-care system becomes involved (Hofland 1992), most particularly fear of being placed (Hood 1987, Rogers & Holm 1994, Tideiksaar 1994). This is a valid concern, particularly in Canada with its high rate of institutionalisation (Forbes et al 1987). Incontinence frequently strains relationships with family caregivers and so leads to placement (Walsh et al 1989), and falls are a leading cause of institutionalisation (Tideiksaar 1994). Both incontinence (Hood 1987, Walsh et al 1989) and elder abuse (McDonald et al 1995) are sources of shame and social isolation, and abuse victims may fear reprisals if they report the abuse (McDonald et al 1995). Pain appears to be underreported because many older adults have internalised the ageist view that pain is a part of normal ageing and must simply be tolerated (Hofland 1992). Similarly, many older adults believe that ill health is a part of normal ageing, and thus they may see themselves as relatively healthy (Clarke 1987) rather than seeking out health care.

Client-centred strategies: therapeutic use of self

Trust is identified as a foundation for therapeutic relationships (Canadian Association of Occupational Therapists 1991). Many older adults may be predisposed to trust health professionals, although they may trust older professionals more than younger ones (Hofland 1992). Nevertheless, an unusually high level of trust may be needed to ensure that the client is not underreporting significant health problems that can and should be addressed in therapy. By conscious therapeutic use of self, the therapist can demonstrate trustworthiness so that the client is more apt to report health status accurately and enter into the sort of honest partnership that client-centred care requires.

Particularly during the assessment phase of therapy, the older client may suffer a higher level of anxiety than a younger one (Edelstein & Semenchuk 1996). Potential reasons for this include more rapid fatigue during the assessment process, the need to share intimate information, frustration about difficulty answering some questions, and recognition of failing memory (Edelstein & Semenchuk 1996). This author has also observed that clients with low levels of formal education particularly fear standardised assessments and frequently depreciate themselves and their abilities before ever attempting the task. The therapist must deliberately establish a relaxed assessment atmosphere where the client dares to participate in the assessment process and wherein the client is relaxed enough to perform optimally (Edelstein & Semenchuk 1996). This can be facilitated by communicating confidence in the client's capacity to improve in response to treatment (Kiernat 1991).

Another method for fostering trust is to debunk some of the common fears held by older clients. Openly telling the client that many clients underreport specific problems, and why, is a start. Clients often fear that their problems are unique, especially such stigmatised ones as incontinence and elder abuse. It is important to go on to explain the adverse consequences of underreporting, that the problems are not addressed and may become worse, as well as the benefit of full disclosure, that a solution can be sought. Clients may fear that there is no solution to their problem or that the only solution is one they dread. Therapists who suspect a particular problem should outline several potential solutions so that the client begins to understand that there are more attractive options. Clients are far more likely to open up if they believe that counselling is an option for the family member who is abusing them than if they believe that the only recourse is court action. Likewise clients are more apt to report falls if the outcome may be environmental modification to their own home rather than removal to a nursing home. Clients need the reassurance that less drastic measures will always be explored first.

Life experience

It has been said that people are the products of their upbringing and experiences. Older clients bring a lifetime of experiences to the therapeutic relationship. They have a long history of facing life's challenges, which may have enhanced their coping strategies (Turk-Charles et al 1996). They may also have a lifetime of habits that may be difficult to change, although Kiernat (1991) argues that such habits are efficient. Many older adults have had vastly different life experiences than most of their much younger health-care providers, specifically personal experience of the Great Depression and of World War II. Some clients may also bring attitudes no longer widely accepted, including racial intolerance and strongly differentiated sex roles. Client-centred practice requires a respect for diversity (Law et al 1995), even when therapist and client values diverge.

Many older clients also come to therapy with experiences in the role of patient. Clients may assume a passive role in the health-care relationship because that is what was previously expected of them. The traditional medical model of care invests the physician with authority over the patient (Barris et al 1988). With this as the basis of their experience, older clients may be surprised or alarmed when asked to assume a decision-making role in their care, even questioning the professional's skills or knowledge level.

Client-centred strategies: education and client control

Therapists must not assume that clients know what their responsibilities are in a client-centred relationship, much less that they are confident about their ability to assume them or are even willing to try to do so. Therapists learn how to practise in a client-centred manner. Likewise, clients need to learn how to participate in client-centred care, especially as this may be significantly different from their previous experiences in health care. It is the responsibility of the therapist to teach them. Specific suggestions for this were discussed earlier in the chapter. However, during the education process, or if the client is adamant about not wishing to assume the degree of responsibility inherent in the client-centred therapeutic partnership, the therapist may need to allow the client to moderate the degree of client centredness to one he or she finds acceptable.

CONCLUSION

Entire books are written about the treatment of the elderly; this chapter is only trying to focus on using a client-centred approach with elderly people. This approach requires that therapists 'determine who the client is [and] respect the client's value system and culture' (Law et al 1995, p. 254). To that end, this chapter has considered the typical life circumstances of older adults, some unique factors influencing their health status, and the attitudes that may be held by both the older client and the health practitioner that may present barriers to client-centred care with older adults. There are many ways to overcome these barriers and facilitate client-centred care. Six approaches discussed in this chapter are enhanced communication, advocacy, therapeutic use of self, client education, promotion of self-efficacy and client choice, even over the degree of client control. Client-centred practice mandates that the therapist respect the client's decisions. Some older clients may prefer a largely therapist-driven plan of care, and a client-centred therapist must respect that choice.

It is essential to note that this chapter can consider only what is usual among the elderly, but the essence of the client-centred approach is to recognise the individuality of the client. Armed with some information on the typical, it is now up to readers to determine to what extent, if any, this is applicable to each older client whom they treat.

REFERENCES

Abler R M, Fretz B R 1988 Self-efficacy and competence in independent living among oldest old persons. Journal of Gerontology 43(4):S138–S143

Age Concern England 1997 http://www.ace.org.uk/stats

Andrews K 1987 Rehabilitation of the older adult. Edward Arnold, London

Angus D 1991 Caring communities: highlights of the symposium on social supports. Minister of Supply and Services Canada, Ottawa

Bandura A 1978 Self-efficacy: toward a unifying theory of behavioral change. Advanced Behavioral Research and Therapy 1:139–161

Bandura A, Adams N E 1977 Analysis of self-efficacy theory of behavioral change. Cognitive Therapy and Research 1(4):287–310

Barris R, Kielhofner G, Watts J H 1988 The medical model. In: Kielhofner G (ed) Bodies of knowledge in psychosocial practice. Slack, Thorofare, New Jersey, ch 1, pp 3–16

Bonder B R 1994 Growing old in the United States. In: Bonder B R, Wagner M B (eds) Functional performance in older adults. F A Davis, Philadelphia, ch 1, pp 4–14

Brummel-Smith K 1990 Introduction. In: Kemp B, Brummel-Smith K, Ramsdell J W (eds) Geriatric rehabilitation. College-Hill, Boston, ch 1, pp 3–21

Canadian Association of Occupational Therapists 1991 Occupational therapy guidelines for client-centred practice. Canadian Association of Occupational Therapists, Toronto

Chernoff R 1996 Nutritional rehabilitation and the elderly. In: Lewis C B (ed) Aging: the health care challenge. F A Davis, Philadelphia, ch 13, pp 305–324

Clarke J 1987 The paradoxical effects of aging on health. Journal of Gerontological Social Work 10(3/4):3–20

Cooper B A 1985 A model for implementing color contrast in the environment for the elderly. American Journal of Occupational Therapy 39(4):253–258

Davis C M 1996 Psychosocial aspects of aging. In: Lewis C B (ed) Aging: the health care challenge. F A Davis, Philadelphia, ch 2, pp 18–44

Dychtwald K, Flower J 1990 Age wave: the challenges and opportunities of an aging America. Bantam, New York

Edelstein B A, Semenchuk E M 1996 Interviewing older adults. In: Carstensen L L, Edelstein B A, Dornbrand L (eds) The practical handbook of clinical gerontology. Sage, Thousand Oaks, California, ch 7, pp 153–173

Forbes W F, Jackson J A, Kraus A S 1987 Institutionalization of the elderly in Canada. Butterworths, Toronto

Galanos A N, Strauss R P, Pieper C F 1994 Sociodemographic correlates of health beliefs among black and white community dwelling elderly individuals. International Journal of Aging and Human Development 38(4):339–350

Helm M 1987 Theories of ageing and current attitudes to old age. In: Helm M (ed) Occupational therapy with the elderly. Churchill Livingstone, Edinburgh, ch 1, pp 10–15

Hofland S L 1992 Elder beliefs: blocks to pain management. Journal of Gerontological Nursing 18(6):19–24

Hood N 1987 Urinary incontinence. In: Helm M (ed) Occupational therapy with the elderly. Churchill Livingstone, Edinburgh, ch 14, pp 147–158

Kielhofner G 1985 A model of human occupation: theory and application. Williams & Wilkins, Baltimore

Kiernat J M 1991 The rewards and challenges of working with older adults. In: Kiernat J M (ed) Occupational therapy and the older adult: a clinical manual. Aspen, Gaithersburg, Maryland, ch 1, pp 2–10

Kolanowski A M 1992 The clinical importance of environmental lighting to the elderly. Journal of Gerontological Nursing 18(1):10–14

Lai S 1990 Living with sensory loss: hearing (NACA writings in gerontology). Minister of Supply and Services Canada, Ottawa

Law M, Baptiste S, Mills J 1995 Client-centred practice: what does it mean and does it make a difference? Canadian Journal of Occupational Therapy 62(5):250–257

Law M, Polatajko H, Baptiste S, Townsend E 1997 Core concepts in occupational therapy. In: Canadian Association of Occupational Therapists (ed) Enabling occupation: an occupational therapy perspective. Canadian Association of Occupational Therapists, Ottawa, ch 3, pp 29–56

Lawton M P 1985 The elderly in context: perspectives from environmental psychology and gerontology. Environment and Behavior 17(4):501–519

Lawton M P, Nahemow L 1973 Ecology and the aging process. In: Eisdorfer C, Lawton M P (eds) The psychology of adult development and aging. American Psychological Association, Washington, DC, pp 619–674

Levy L L 1986 Sensory change and compensation. In: Davis LJ, Kirkland M (eds) The role of occupational therapy with the elderly. American Occupational Therapy Association, Rockville, Maryland, pp 49–67

McDonald L, Pittaway E, Nahmiash D 1995 Issues in practice with respect to mistreatment of older people. In: MacLean M J (ed) Abuse and neglect of older Canadians: strategies for change. Thompson, Toronto, ch 1-1, pp 5–16

Minister of National Health and Welfare 1993 Aging and independence: overview of a national survey. Minister of Supply and Services Canada, Ottawa

Naeyaert K 1990 Living with sensory loss: vision (NACA Writings in Gerontology). Minister of Supply and Services Canada, Ottawa

National Advisory Council on Aging 1990 Informal caregiving: support and enhancement. Minister of Supply and Services Canada, Ottawa

National Advisory Council on Aging 1991 The economic situation of Canada's seniors. Minister of Supply and Services Canada, Ottawa

National Advisory Council on Aging 1993a Aging vignette #1 – how many? Men vs. women? How old? All married? National Advisory Council on Aging, Ottawa

National Advisory Council on Aging 1993b Aging vignette #6 – how healthy? For how long? National Advisory Council on Aging, Ottawa

National Advisory Council on Aging 1993c Aging vignette #11 – Needing support for daily living? From whom? National Advisory Council on Aging, Ottawa

National Advisory Council on Aging 1995 Community services in health care for seniors: progress and challenges. Minister of Supply and Services Canada, Ottawa.

National Advisory Council on Aging 1996 Aging vignette #54 – a quick portrait of Canada's retirement income system. National Advisory Council on Aging, Ottawa

Novak M 1993 Aging and society: a Canadian perspective. Nelson, Scarborough, Ontario

Office of Gerontological Studies 1996 Facts on aging in Canada. McMaster University, Hamilton, Ontario

Orange J B, Ryan E B 1995 Effective communication. In: Pickles B, Compton A, Cott C, Simpson J, Vandervoort A (eds) Physiotherapy with older people. W B Saunders, London, ch 10, pp 119–137

Rogers C R 1951 Client-centred therapy: its current practice, implications, and theory. Houghton Mifflin, Boston

Rogers J C, Holm M B 1994 Assessment of self-care. In: Bonder B R, Wagner M B (eds) Functional performance in older adults. F A Davis, Philadelphia, ch 12, pp 181–202

Ross N P, Shapiro E, Roos L L Jr 1984 Aging and the demand for health services: which aged and whose demand? Gerontologist 24(1):31–36

Schwenger C W, Gross M J 1980 Institutional care and institutionalization of the elderly in Canada. In: Marchall V W (ed) Aging in Canada. Fitzhenry & Whiteside, Don Mills, Ontario, ch 23, pp 248–256

Shilton M 1995 Attitudes toward ageing and older people. In: Pickles B, Compton A, Cott C, Simpson S, Vandervoort A (eds) Physiotherapy with older people. W B Saunders, London, ch 3, pp 29–42

Stone L O, DeWit M 1991 Association between uses of formal and informal sources of support in help received

by the older population. In: Angus D (ed) Caring communities: highlights of the symposium on social supports. Minister of Supply and Services Canada, Ottawa, p 36

Stone R, Cafferata G L, Sangl J 1987 Caregivers of the frail elderly: a national profile. Gerontologist 27(5):616–626

Strain L A 1989 Illness behaviours in old age. Journal of Aging Studies 3(4):325–340

Thorson J A, Powell F C 1991 Age differences in health attitudes and beliefs. Psychological Reports 69:1111–1115

Tideiksaar R 1994 Falls. In: Bonder B R, Wagner M B (eds) Functional performance in older adults. F A Davis, Philadelphia, ch 14, pp 224–239

Tobias J S, Block M, Steinhaus-Donham C, Reinsch S, Tamaru K, Weil D 1990 Falling among the sensorially impaired elderly. Archives of Physical Medicine and Rehabilitation 71:144–147

Todd A K, Rider B A, Page-Robin E 1986 Attitudes of occupational therapy students toward older persons. Physical and Occupational Therapy in Geriatrics 5(2):71–81

Turk-Charles S, Rose T, Gatz M 1996 The significance of gender in the treatment of older adults. In: Carstensen L L, Edelstein B A, Dornbrand L (eds) The practical handbook of clinical gerontology. Sage, Thousand Oaks, California, ch 5, pp 107–128

van Maanen HMTh 1988 Being old does not always mean being sick: perspectives of health as perceived by British and American elderly. Journal of Advanced Nursing 13:701–709

Waller K V, Bates R C 1992 Health locus of control and self-efficacy beliefs in a healthy elderly sample. American Journal of Health Promotion 6(4):303–309

Walsh J R, Tsukuda R A W, Miller J 1989 Management of the frail elderly by the health care team. Green, St Louis

Waxler-Morrison N 1990 Introduction. In: Waxler-Morrison N, Anderson J, Richardson E (eds) Cross-cultural caring: a handbook for health professionals. University of British Columbia Press, Vancouver, ch 1, pp 3–10

Yee B W K, Williams B J 1996 Medication management and appropriate substance use for the elderly. In: Lewis C B (ed) Aging: the health care challenge. F A Davis, Philadelphia, ch 14, pp 325–363

Zeiss A M, Steffen A M 1996 Interdisciplinary health care teams: the basic unit of geriatric care. In: Carstensen L L, Edelstein B A, Dornbrand L (eds) The practical handbook of clinical gerontology. Sage, Thousand Oaks, California, ch 19, pp 423–450

8

The challenges of client-centred practice in mental health settings

A. Kusznir
E. Scott

This chapter reviews the development of client-centred practice in psychiatric occupational therapy and, by means of case studies, highlights some of the common challenges to the maintenance of a client-centred approach in mental health settings. Therapists may, at certain junctures, need to be directive; optimal management of this departure from client centredness represents a significant challenge.

Despite the benefits and rewards to both the client and therapist, working in a client-centred model of practice in mental health settings is both challenging and complex. For many occupational therapists, the incorporation of a client-centred approach may appear initially effortless, as many therapists are less entrenched in a traditional medical model than many of their colleagues. Additionally, many occupational therapists already practise in a client-focused model of care such as psychosocial rehabilitation. Few therapists, however, are left feeling that their efforts to maintain a client-centred focus in their practice have never been challenged.

The purpose of this chapter is to review the development of client-centred practice in psychiatric occupational therapy as well as to outline and discuss some of the common challenges that threaten an adherence to a client-centred framework in everyday practice in mental health settings. Included in the discussion will be recommendations for practice that represent the collective opinion of nine experienced mental health occupational therapists employed at a psychiatric research and clinical facility, the Centre for

Addiction and Mental Health – Clarke Division, in Toronto, Canada.

THE DEVELOPMENT OF CLIENT-CENTRED PRACTICE IN MENTAL HEALTH

Under the auspices of the Canadian Association of Occupational Therapists (CAOT), occupational therapists in Canada have worked to develop and operationalise client-centred practice guidelines for more than 15 years. The early efforts of CAOT included the development of generic guidelines describing the stages of occupational therapy practice applicable to a wide range of practice settings. The foundation of these early generic guidelines formed the basis of a client-centred approach to occupational therapy services in Canada (Department of National Health and Welfare & CAOT 1983). These guidelines have been widely distributed and used in Canada (Blain & Townsend 1993) and the term 'client-centred' has found a common place in the lexicon of many Canadian occupational therapists.

In 1993, CAOT in cooperation with Health Canada refined these earlier generic guidelines with the publication of a document entitled *Occupational therapy guidelines for client-centred mental health practice*. In this document client-centred practice is broadened from the philosophical orientation of respect and partnership to a definition emphasising a collaborative relationship between the client and therapist. Client knowledge and experiences are primary. The therapist's attention to the client's verbal and non-verbal cues for an understanding of the client's definition of purposeful and meaningful occupational performance is seen as a critical component of this collaborative relationship (CAOT 1993).

The document further defines some of the parameters and functions of the therapist and client in this collaboration. Specifically, it is recommended that the therapist actively seek out and structure opportunities for choices and decisions that are commensurate with the client's skills and experiences. Clients are encouraged to develop the requisite skills and roles to participate in their own assessment, planning and intervention. Furthermore, the occupational therapist has a moral and ethical responsibility to ensure that clients are informed of the possible options and risks connected with a particular course of treatment and/or action. The authors also recognise that this emphasis on client choice, authority, risk-taking and a spirit of equality within the client–therapist relationship demands an organisational system that acknowledges a client's abilities, and shares the ethical, moral and legal responsibility for their decisions (CAOT 1993).

The most recent refinement of the client-centred framework can be found in the development of core concepts of the Canadian Model of Occupational Performance as outlined in *Enabling occupation: an occupational therapy perspective* (CAOT 1997). Although this document does not focus exclusively on practice within mental health settings, one of the core occupational therapy values and beliefs about client-centred practice includes the belief that clients have experience and knowledge about their occupation; that clients are active partners in the occupational therapy process; risk-taking is necessary for positive change; and that client-centred practice in occupational therapy focuses on enabling occupation. More importantly, the Canadian Model of Occupational Performance illustrates the connection between a person's engagement in meaningful occupations and the interaction with an environment, and how occupational therapy's philosophy of client-centred practice is translated into practice through the processes of enablement.

Enablement differs from treatment, as it not only involves the client as an active participant in the occupational therapy process, but also involves the process of 'facilitating, guiding, coaching, educating, prompting, listening, reflecting, encouraging or otherwise collaborating with people so that individuals, groups, agencies, or organizations have the means and opportunity to participate in shaping their own lives' (CAOT 1997, p. 50). Client-centred practice is defined as a collaborative approach aimed at 'enabling occupation with clients who may be individuals, groups, agencies, governments, corporations or others'. Central to this approach is respect for clients, involving the acknowledgement of their experience and knowledge, clients' involvement in decision-making, and advocating with and for clients in meeting their needs (CAOT 1997, p. 49).

There are several other significant contributions to the development of a client-centred focus in mental health practice for occupational therapists. Many other scholars and educators of occupational therapy (Bruce and Christiansen 1988, Yerxa 1994) maintain that, since the first days of the profession, occupational therapists have endorsed a humanistic philosophy that values individual choice and the right to self-fulfilment. The American Occupational Therapy Association's identification of seven core values underlying the profession also reflect the spirit of client-centred practice. Implicit in the core values of altruism, equality, freedom, justice, dignity, truth and prudence (AOTA 1993) is not only a focus on humanistic ideals, but also on working with clients in a caring and therapeutic relationship.

The qualitative investigations of the components of therapeutic rapport that followed and supported the identification of the above seven core values contribute to the understanding of client-centred practice. Devereaux (1984) highlighted how caring forms the fundamental ingredient in the evolution of a therapeutic relationship, and how connecting with clients is pivotal in helping clients maintain their optimal level of occupational performance. Peloquin (1995), in her examination and reflection on empathy, provided an examination of the client–therapist relationship and concluded that 'competence and caring' are critical to the establishment of a collaborative relationship. Peloquin (1990) also provided a review of unhelpful encounters between clients and their caregivers that highlight how issues of power and dispassionate behaviour can negatively influence a collaborative and therapeutic relationship.

Rosa and Hasselkus (1996) explored the characteristics of collaborative therapeutic relationships in a qualitative study examining the personal experiences of 83 therapists connecting with their clients. The investigators interviewed therapists across several specialty areas in an effort to describe the therapists' perceptions of clients in relationships described as 'working together' versus 'not working together'. The narratives detailing the sense of joining together in a mutually supportive partnership usually involved a client whom the therapist perceived as 'motivated, hardworking, determined, fun to work with, appreciative and even inspiring.' The 'not helping' and 'not working together' relationships usually included a therapist making unrealistic recommendations and having little opportunity and time to develop a therapeutic relationship with the client. The clients in these relationships were often viewed as having an angry or depressed disposition, a poor understanding of occupational therapy, a complaint about lack of progress of treatment, or a negative reaction toward the therapist which, on rare occasions, included physical assault. Needless to say, most occupational therapists in mental health settings have at one point in their career come close to experiencing some if not all of these unfortunate scenarios.

Occupational therapists in mental health settings are often faced with a unique set of challenges when they are asked to participate in non-treatment, professional collaborations with people with mental health disabilities. Haiman (1995) explored some of the dilemmas in professional collaborations that emerged when she joined an education and advocacy project ostensibly aimed at educating potential employers about the employability of people with mental health disabilities. She describes several pertinent scenarios that detail the dilemmas involved in maintaining professional boundaries in various non-treatment scenarios, and concludes that there are no correct answers in handling these boundary dilemmas. Instead, she reflects on the importance of a thoughtful, well-reasoned response that embodies many of the critical components of a client-centred approach. Specifically, she advocates for a caring and holistic approach where there is a respect for a person's identity and a shift in power and authority.

Critical, when reflecting on the development of client-centred practice in mental health, is the contribution of occupational therapists as case managers within the psychosocial rehabilitation model. Krupa and Clark (1995) advocate for the unique and significant role that occupational therapists have as case managers in the delivery of services for persons with severe and persistent psychiatric disorders. Highlighted in their discussion is the relevance of a client-centred approach to service delivery to the implicit and imperative components of case management. These authors also identify that clients' increase in control over the development, implementation and evaluation of services has been advocated by several sources outside the occupational therapy literature (Everett & Nelson 1992, Nikkel et al 1992, Paulson 1991).

Everett & Nelson (1992) provided an interesting description of the evolution of a successful client-centred relationship in which the case manager evolved as an effective partner in the therapeutic process. The client in this relationship was a person with a diagnosis of borderline personality disorder, who presented with threats of self-harm in dealing with her abusive background and a history of substance abuse. The case manager's assumption that the client was a competent adult, despite some of the initial threats by the client of self-harm, emerged as critical in this relationship. Interacting with the client on an 'adult-to-adult basis' was identified as being particularly helpful, as was 'never telling her what to do' and really hearing what she had to say. The authors provide some useful practice guidelines in working with persons with borderline personality disorder that operationalize the philosophy of a client-centred approach. Specifically, transforming the standard psychosocial assessment into a more participatory, user friendly, evaluation was seen as particularly helpful in giving the client a sense of authority and involvement in the initial stages of this therapeutic collaboration.

Along with Everett and Nelson, there are several professional groups outside the discipline of occupational therapy who have embraced the concerns that arise in working within a client-centred approach. Other professional groups, although not always specific to mental health settings, suggest conducting an open and direct evaluation of the relevance of a client-focused approach. In their qualitative indepth interviews of case managers working with the frail elderly, Clemens and colleagues (1994) investigated the extent to which client-centred theory is reflected in case management practice. Case managers identified in this study who were either social workers or nurses endorsed the importance of client-centred theory when working in long-term care settings with the frail and elderly. The investigators identified several themes when a departure from a client-centred philosophy was reported in everyday practice. These themes include the disparity between client wishes and the constraints of the system, the inevitability of a nursing home placement, and the process of adhering to and involving clients in a care plan. Although there is often justification for this departure from a client-centred approach, the authors also advocate the need to address burnout and role conflict which were identified in this study.

Rothman et al (1996) described how social workers are often caught between client self-determination and outcome-oriented, competency-based practice. The investigators conducted a survey of 35 experienced social workers who were asked to provide vignettes illustrating the range of directiveness they used with clients. The results indicate that, although social workers seem to prefer non-directive styles, their practice repertoires include a broad range of directive responses. Moreover, when they reviewed the scenarios where a directive response (i.e. use of an independent action by the practitioner on behalf of a client or client group without their knowledge or acquiescence) was used they determined that it was ethically acceptable in 95% of the cases. Some 86% of the practitioners identified using at least one directive response. The prescriptive model involving the consideration of a problem with a client or client group in which the practitioner clearly indicates a specific course of action was found most problematic ethically.

Advocating for the incorporation of counselling into nursing practice, Burnard (1995) recommended 'client-centred' counselling along with the provision of advice, information and suggestions. Moreover, he advocated striking a balance between sharing of certain experiences with clients to develop autonomy and leaving clients entirely to their own devices. Burnard argued that the client-centred approach bears some inherent theoretical flaws and he is firm in his belief that eschewing all advice-giving removes an important option in the range of counselling possibilities and forces the client to be alone in making a decision. A similar debate is offered by Wilshaw (1997), who discusses the benefits and limitations of adopting a cognitive behavioural versus client-centred approach in mental health nursing. In examining the various factors underlying an effective therapeutic relationship, the author concludes that some flexibility of theoretical affiliation is critical if a mental health nurse is to embrace client-centred practice.

A review of the literature reveals a steady advancement of the theory of client-centred practice within occupational therapy in mental health over the past 15 years. Although occupational therapists can draw on the supporting evidence from the qualitative studies conducted by Peloquin (1990), Rosa and Hasselkus (1996), as well as Devereaux (1984), a more systematic and rigorous approach to evaluating the presence and effectiveness of a client-centred approach in everyday practice is needed. Other professional groups have also embraced client-centred practice and, more importantly, have attempted to assess the extent and limitations of the approach. Although the evaluation of the effectiveness of a client-centred approach in everyday practice is both daunting and necessary, the first step may be to ask therapists in mental health settings for case examples and their perceptions of the challenges to client-centred practice.

INVESTIGATING THE CHALLENGES OF CLIENT-CENTRED PRACTICE IN MENTAL HEALTH

A group of nine occupational therapists at the Centre for Addiction and Mental Health – Clarke Division, working in a wide range of settings with clients with varied mental health problems and age groups, was engaged in a process of identifying the challenges to practising within a client-centred framework. Although each therapist acknowledged a familiarity and embodiment of a client-centred focus, there was also an acknowledgement that this effort was not without its challenges and dilemmas. The process included the submission of case examples typifying the challenges to client-centred practice in mental health settings. In some cases, therapists offered composite cases to illustrate their concerns.

Therapists were also asked to reflect on the specific juncture at which their efforts to maintain a client-centred focus was challenged and to reflect on the outcome of the occupational therapy process. Additionally, therapists were asked to determine whether the outcome was viewed as either positive or negative by both the client and therapist. The case studies were analysed thematically by the authors, and the emergent themes were reviewed for agreement by each therapist. The authors refined recommendations offered in each case by reflecting on the guiding principles for client-centred practice outlined in *Enabling occupation: an occupational therapy perspective* (CAOT 1997). Although the challenges in adhering to a client-centred focus were not restricted to any one stage of care within a mental health setting, the following junctures in the occupational therapy process were identified as particular challenges to client-centred practice:

- client's reluctance to engage in the occupational therapy process
- disagreement in opinion(s) and/or expectation(s) between therapist and client
- client difficulty in making decisions
- lack of fit between client decision and client skill level
- difficulty in modifying the client's environment.

Client's reluctance to engage in the occupational therapy process

Despite the setting, reason for referral or length of involvement, the client's reluctance to engage in the occupational therapy process can be a challenge to client-centred practice. Very often, therapists employed in a short-term stay crisis unit have little opportunity to develop a therapeutic rapport with their clients. Needless to say, the first encounter with a client on a short-stay inpatient unit is critical not only to developing therapeutic rapport but also to engaging the client in the occupational therapy process. This first meeting is an important juncture where a client-centred focus can be challenged.

Take the case of Larry, a 34-year-old single unemployed man with the diagnosis of schizo-affective disorder admitted to an inpatient short-stay unit for stabilization of his medication. Before hospitalisation, Larry was living alone in a bachelor apartment and supporting himself on public assistance. He was of great concern to his older siblings and parents because of his reported difficulty with independent living. According to family reports, he had not washed any dishes or done any laundry for at least a month before his admission. In the initial interview with the occupational therapist, Larry presented as a shy, vague, confused man who questioned the need for a functional assessment. He minimised his family's concerns, stating 'they are just a bunch of neat freaks.' Larry was eager to return to living in his apartment to care for his tropical fish, and insisted that there was little need for a functional assessment as 'things always get done when they are finished.'

The therapist determined the type of activities that were meaningful for Larry and, more important, the type of activities that were of limited value to him, such as cleaning his apartment and completing a functional assessment. The challenge at this juncture was persuading Larry to do something that he did not value or want to do.

Recommendations

- Although it is critical at this point to empathise and reflect on the client's concern, the therapist should be direct in sharing her responsibilities, thereby engaging Larry in the assessment process. Externalising the request for the assessment as being outside

the therapeutic relationship can be very effective.
- Emphasising a collaborative spirit of exploring Larry's strengths, and an impartial attitude about his limitations, can also be helpful.

A client's reluctance to engage in the occupational therapy process can also be seen in other aspects of health-care delivery. After an unsuccessful outcome in resuming employment after a motor vehicle accident, Edward, a 37-year-old man previously employed in various accounting jobs, was referred for an occupational therapy assessment by his insurance company. At the time of his accident, Edward sustained a rotator cuff injury and minor concussion. There were no immediate signs of any brain injury. Although surgery and therapy improved his rotator cuff injury, he started experiencing problems with memory and concentration.

An occupational therapy assessment, along with a psychological evaluation, was requested to determine the need for cognitive remediation and to confirm the presence of any permanent brain damage. In the initial interview, Edward presented as being quite discouraged and angry with the 'insurance system' and their request for yet another assessment. He viewed the assessment as an invasion of his privacy, and focused on externalising the difficulties he had had with his bosses in the few minor work assignments he had obtained since the accident. Regardless, his anger and passive acceptance to participate in the assessment process presented as a challenge to the focus on a client-centred approach.

Recommendations

- By giving the client the opportunity to vent his concerns, the therapist could identify the underlying impairments in Edward's mood and affect. While further questioning revealed that he was experiencing an episode of major depression, the challenge of engaging Edward in a process into which he felt forced needed to be addressed.

• The therapist's effort to empower Edward by emphasising and providing information about the consequences of his choice of not participating in the assessment may be helpful. The therapist could also give Edward choices in the order of administration of the assessment modalities.

Edward became less hostile and resistant to completing the assessment and by the end of the evaluation he expressed his appreciation for the therapist's understanding and explanations. Additionally Edward was able to develop an understanding of the potential impact of depression, and ultimately the reason for his impaired work performance.

Added challenges to client-centred practice can be seen when the client initiates the occupational therapy process. Cindy was a 38-year-old single woman, self-employed in the adult entertainment field. Although quite pessimistic about any benefit from psychiatry, she sought a referral to an outpatient mental health clinic to deal with her depression. After her second session with the psychiatrist, she had shared her desire to secure alternative employment. Although she had also shared her sense of shame and the allure of being in such a high-paying occupation, she appeared interested in vocational counselling.

Cindy was seen for two sessions by the outpatient occupational therapist, where she briefly reviewed her life story and detailed some of her concerns about her current occupation. Cindy did not follow up with her third and fourth appointments, even though she had expressed an interest in the therapist's proposed goals of completing interest surveys and reviewing some written information on stress management. Despite the therapist's effort to review Cindy's occupational history in an informal and non-judgemental manner, Cindy declined further involvement in an occupational therapy process. When questioned by her psychiatrist, Cindy expressed a concern that she was letting her therapist down, and stated that she may consider involvement at a later date. Although, in retrospect, Cindy's involvement in occupational therapy was premature, there

were no indications of these concerns in any of the sessions.

Recommendations

• Helping the client to understand her response and reactions to the occupational therapy process is imperative. It was very important that the therapist met with the client to discuss her decision to discontinue her involvement in occupational therapy and reassure her that she had the right to make that decision. Guiding the client to identify her own needs was critical in maintaining a client-centred focus.

To date, although Cindy is continuing with her individual therapy, she has not requested a return to work with the occupational therapist.

Disagreement in opinion(s) and/or expectation(s) between therapist and client

Although the client's experiences and knowledge are paramount in client-centred practice and carry authority in the client–professional partnership, this does not negate the importance of professional expertise (CAOT 1993). Challenges to client-centred practice emerge when professional expertise or opinion conflicts with clients' opinions or concerns about their abilities, the course of treatment or programming. Occupational therapists can easily address this challenge when the issue of risk is obvious, but in a mental health setting the issue of risk is often more speculative and less distinct.

The case of Jane, a 45-year-old unemployed woman with a diagnosis of bipolar disorder, can illustrate this point. Although Jane had not worked in 5 years, she had been employed as a cashier for 17 years. She left this job when she inherited a sizeable inheritance, but was admitted almost destitute as she had squandered this money while in a manic state. Unwilling to secure employment as a cashier, Jane was referred to occupational therapy to review her occupational options. A brief functional assessment revealed that she exhibited significant problems in the components of occupational performance required for competitive employment. Although Jane acknowledged that she had problems with her concentration and memory, she insisted that she needed to secure paid employment to recover her debts. Although Jane did not agree with the recommendation that she was not ready for work, and that a rehabilitation and/or training programme was a more suitable option, she did agree to continued contact with the therapist over the next few months while job searching. Additionally, the therapist and client were able to set goals with respect to the length of time she would be job searching before she would consider enrolment in rehabilitation training programmes. Sanctioning the client's effort to job search facilitated this goal-setting process.

Recommendations

- Empathising with the client's concern that she wanted to regain her financial losses was helpful for maintaining follow-up with Jane. The individual follow-up sessions were also helpful to assess any risks and follow her progress in her job search.
- Being direct but tactful in outlining any disagreements between therapist and client is important. Additionally, the therapist needs to outline clearly the rationale for any decisions and in language understandable to the client.

Jane is continuing her job search and remains unwilling to consider any training and/or rehabilitation options. She has adjusted to supporting herself on public assistance, and despite her difficulty in getting up in the morning, has applied for work about once a week.

In cases where the opportunity to monitor a client's progress is not feasible, the occupational therapist in conjunction with his or her team members needs to outline the risks more directly and plan for the possibility of failure. A useful example can be seen with Martha, an 81-year-old widowed and retired school teacher living alone in a large two-storey home. Martha was admitted to hospital with a broken leg and arm after a

fall in her home. In hospital, she presented with declining mental status, in particular a poor memory along with symptoms of depression and rheumatoid arthritis. After making an adequate physical recovery, she was transferred to a geriatric psychiatric unit to address her problems with her mood and memory as well as to prepare for discharge. Her mood quickly improved with the occupational therapist's effort to include her in various social and therapeutic groups. Martha revealed herself to be a bright and sociable individual who was quite adamant about returning to live in her own home. Meeting her social needs seemed critical in warding off any problems with depression.

The occupational therapist was asked to assess Martha's capacity for independent living and make recommendations for discharge. Her physical injuries had left her dependent on a walker and unable to perform many activities of daily living. The decreased range of motion in her upper extremities also made it very difficult for her to dress independently. Although she could make herself a cup of tea, she had difficulty with more complex food preparation tasks. Problems with fatigue and balance were also apparent, as she needed support to climb stairs. A home visit revealed that Martha lived in a large home that was in considerable disrepair. There were no lights working in the entire home because she could not change any light bulbs. Although this partially explained her fall, several other concerns became evident. With the placement of her furniture, Martha could not use her walker in her home. She was quite proud, however, that she could 'furniture crawl'. Martha was not particularly discouraged about being confined to the first level of her home.

Despite Martha's conviction to stay in her home, a nursing home was the most logical conclusion for Martha's family and many of her treatment team members. The occupational therapist undertook the effort to advocate on Martha's behalf and make arrangements to convert her first floor to include a bathroom. Despite the myriad of community supports that were put in place, several significant problems soon became apparent. With no one to assist Martha in dressing in the evenings, the option of sleeping in her day clothes became inevitable. Exploration of this option with Martha revealed that she remained resolute and unperturbed about the option of sleeping in her clothes, as long as she could stay in her own home.

Recommendations

- Understanding and respecting a client's own style of coping and adapting to demands was needed. This process requires providing the client with choices that may not necessarily reflect the therapist's or the treatment team's values.
- In working with team members it is important to emphasise the importance of client values and choices. Many staff members working with Martha were concerned about the prospect of her living independently, and failed to see that independent living was the only option that she valued.
- Although the authors are reminded of the work by Clemens and colleagues (1994), and the inevitability of nursing home placement for many frail and elderly individuals, focusing on what the client wanted to do, rather than what she could do, was critical in maintaining a client-centred focus.

Client difficulty in making decisions

Within a client-centred framework the client carries the authority to make decisions, but there are times when it is clear that a client is having problems making and staying with a decision. Take the example of Lisa, a 40-year-old elementary school teacher who had been off work for the past 3 years. She had developed her first episode of major depression after being off sick with a viral infection. When seen in occupational therapy, she presented as being quite tearful, somewhat irritable, as well as bewildered and ashamed of her current condition. She had particular problems with fatigue and decision-making, and was extremely self-critical. Lisa was shown and asked her opinion about a written

report prepared by the therapist and requested by her insurance company. The letter outlined a rehabilitation plan developed by both Lisa and the therapist. Lisa found this request to be quite overwhelming and retorted by expressing concerns about the therapist's expertise and knowledge of such matters.

Recommendations

- It was critical to reflect on the client's struggle with depressive symptoms as a way of helping her to understand her own responses. Interpreting Lisa's difficulty in making a decision as part of her depression, rather than allowing her to compare the depreciation of her skills and abilities, was necessary.
- Every client presents with his or her own threshold for being overwhelmed with practical issues. This threshold is dependent upon the client's experience with various systems, and overall mood and confidence level.

With the improvement of Lisa's depressive symptoms, she was able to gain control and confidence over some of the tasks that concerned her in the home and in her volunteer placement. Although she continues to be perplexed about her lengthy absence from work, she is now actively participating in deciding on the programmes and activities that will help her regain her work capacity.

Sometimes, a client's difficulty in staying with a decision can also create a challenge in maintaining a client-centred focus. An example of this can be seen with Mathew's response to a decision to move into a public-assisted supportive residence. Mathew is a 38-year-old single man with a diagnosis of schizoaffective disorder who was faced with a housing crisis. Because of annual rent increases, he was seeing his public assistance cheque getting smaller each year. Additionally, Mathew felt quite socially isolated and found meal preparation to be quite burdensome. He attended various community programmes that offered daily meals, but remained dissatisfied with the quality of his meals, social contacts and activities. His name had been put on a waiting list for a place in a cooperative living residence for persons with mental health disabilities, and he initially appeared quite excited about the prospects of community living.

After an interview with the staff at the residence, Mathew became somewhat focused on the rules of the residence and the condition of having to leave if there were any signs of inappropriate behaviour or discontinuation of his medication. He was concerned that, should this happen, his only option would be that of homelessness. A conversation with his mother confirmed his concerns and desire to withdraw his application. Despite efforts to explain the cause and criteria for such inappropriate behaviour, as well as reinforcing the opinion that Mathew presents as being a polite and compassionate individual who had been faithfully taking his medication for the past 20 years, he remained convinced that he should not risk moving.

Recommendations

Assessing the source and antecedent of stress affecting the change in the client's opinion and outlook is imperative. In this situation, instead of siding with the client's decision, it was important to recognise that the fear of becoming homeless and the shame associated with this possibility, however remote, was very real for Mathew.

• It was necessary to be directive, by offering to discuss his concerns with his mother and to speak with the resident counsellors.
• Adopting the approach of engaging the client in a process of examining the risks and consequences was minimally helpful once Mathew had become preoccupied with anxiety with regard to the move, and served only to perpetuate his difficulties in making a decision.

Although Matthew continued to feel somewhat overwhelmed by the move, he found such a directive approach by the therapist to be helpful. He is quite satisfied with the social network and supports available in his new residence and acknowledges a dramatic change in the quality of his life.

Lack of fit between client decision and client skill level

Each of the previous case scenarios illustrates a client who made a decision that was within his or her skill or capabilities. Working in mental health settings often brings more complex challenges to client-centred practice, as often there is a lack of fit between clients' decision and their skill level. When Robert was first seen for occupational therapy services, he was a 35-year-old divorced man with a diagnosis of chronic refractory depression. He had previously been employed as a laboratory technician, and decided that retraining to become a stockbroker would help in his overall recovery. While employed, he had dabbled in the market, and found the financial rewards to be quite easy. He recognised, however, that he had made a few poor business decisions which he believed had led not only to the breakup of his marriage, but to the onset of his depression and several lengthy hospitalisations. A thorough educational, vocational and psychological assessment revealed that Robert had a significant learning disability, and that he had significant problems with both spelling and reversal of numbers. Although Robert was directly cautioned that his vocational goal was unrealistic, he was given the opportunity to engage in an upgrading programme while waiting for remedial training. After a year, Robert had made only marginal improvement in his academic skills, but was still fixed in his vocational goal.

Although Robert's contact with occupational therapy was terminated because he would not consider other vocational options, he re-established contact with occupational therapy several years later as he requested some assistance in social skills training and time management. Robert was now enrolled in a course preparing him for the necessary stockbrokers' examinations. He was failing some of his courses, and had specific problems with the required group assignments. He felt that many students avoided him and that he was not getting the help from instructors that he needed. Robert made only minor progress with the individual sessions. He continued to focus on his sense of alienation as a cause of his difficulties. Robert did not pass his course and he remains unwilling to consider alternative job options. The therapist speculates that the initial directive approach motivated Robert to seek out his own resources while the client-centred approach only added to his tendency to externalise his limitations.

Recommendations

- Although it was important for the therapist to maintain an unbiased rapport with the client throughout the occupational therapy process, a client's strong tendency to externalise limitations may evade any positive outcome when there is a lack of fit between client decision and client skill level.

Inevitably there are occasions when occupational therapists in mental health settings are required to be directive while still challenged to maintain a client-centred focus. The efforts to mobilise a group of eight clients in a self-employment initiative is probably the best example of this. The Productivity Plus group included eight members, three men and five women, most of whom had a severe and persistent mental illness of either schizophrenia, schizoaffective disorder or bipolar disorder. All clients had been hospitalised several times and were on medications with mixed and refractory responses. Although most clients had not worked in several years and had unsuccessful experiences in vocational rehabilitation programmes, they still wanted to be employed. Collectively the group determined that they were going to sell their own handicraft sewing projects and met weekly, not only to make their products, but also to plan a strategy for their business.

The purpose of the subsequent groups facilitated by occupational therapy was to create a meaningful and financially rewarding work situation that would enable clients to re-establish hope and confidence in their ability to maintain involvement in meaningful occupation. The therapists also wanted to establish and maintain a sense of community within the group, to provide skills training if necessary and, more importantly, to take direction from clients in order to create and advocate for an environment that would meet the work-related needs of the group of participants. The clients who entered the group wanted not only to work, but also to demonstrate their responsibility and abilities to their family and friends, to make friends and be with friends, and to have their own business.

The most common challenge identified by the therapists in maintaining a client-centred focus was to facilitate the group and/or decision-making process without dominating or leading the group. This was especially challenging when the group was faced with a problem or was needing to make a decision. Additional concerns in maintaining a client-centred focus developed when dealing with the financial profits of the group, encouraging risk-taking and moving the programme outside the hospital and into the community.

With respect to the group process, therapists found that there were multiple and complex expectations and skills that needed to be considered. Specifically, when or how to enable the development of leadership within the group, when to step in to support the work being done, and when not to step in, remained ongoing challenges. Clients volunteered to work at a display table during a craft show. Issues such as how the group dealt with the scheduled person who did not show up to staff the table called for assessing each situation on an individual basis and drawing on experiences of the group. Often the ability to plan and prepare was not a strength of the group members, and the therapists of the group often found themselves at odds with the group consensus. The therapists found that it was critical to create an environment that reflected the wishes of the participants, as comfort and inclusion needed to be balanced with individual skill teaching.

Recommendations

• Although from the onset, the occupational therapists were aligned with the client-centred approach and implemented many of the guiding principles a directive approach was unavoidable, and needed on several occasions.

Today the members of Productivity Plus continue to meet in a community centre and the group continues to be a viable source of supplemental income for all participants. More importantly, the group members now have limited input from the original therapists involved in developing the project.

Difficulty in modifying the client's environment

The Canadian Model of Occupational Performance highlights the interpretation between a person's engagement in meaningful occupations and the environment (CAOT 1997). At times, there are critical and recurring issues in a client's environment that can have a significant impact on the clinical outcome and effort to maintain a client-centred focus. Consider the case of Henry, an 8-year-old presenting with oppositional defiant disorder, panic disorder, school phobia, separation anxiety and attention deficit disorder. Henry is an only child in a two-parent family living on public assistance and in subsidised housing. He required heavy doses of barbiturates to control his violent outbursts, anxiety and inattention.

On admission to a children's day treatment programme, Henry was diagnosed with a severe developmental coordination disorder. When asked to perform age-appropriate tasks, he would become anxious, oppositional and at times violent. Henry worked with the occupational therapist to develop new insights and problem-solving strategies for these everyday tasks. By generating precise goals for mastering climbing stairs, preparing basic foods, being a fair playmate and engaging in community activities, and by working with his parents, Henry was able to generalise his new skills at home and in his community.

Over his 18-month involvement in a day treatment programme, Henry made dramatic improvement in his skills and gained more than 6 years of competence. Upon discharge, he was placed in a specialised classroom programme. With regular liaison with the parents, key school personnel supported Henry's successful reintegration to his community school. However, midway through the year, Henry experienced a series of personal losses (e.g. death of his grandmother, resignation of two favourite teachers) and there was a breakdown of parental supports and communications with school personnel. Henry regressed, and began to experience problems with attention, anxiety and impulse-control.

Recommendations

• Despite adherence to many of the guiding principles of client-centred practice, the importance of considering the transaction of the client in his or her environment cannot be overlooked. A therapist must extend the intervention to advocate for appropriate environmental conditions before a meaningful and positive way can be maintained.

After being expelled from school, Henry was placed in a new treatment setting. However, only after reinvolvement with the original treatment team did his behaviour stabilise.

CONCLUSION

Dealing with the challenges of maintaining a client-centred framework in mental health practice settings requires a sensitivity to clients' needs, moods, values and vision coupled with an acute awareness of the junctures in the occupational therapy process at which adherence to a client-centred focus is threatened. The junctures identified in this chapter include a client's reluctance to engage in the occupational therapy process; a disagreement in opinion(s) and/or expectation(s) between therapist and client; a client's difficulty making a decision; the lack of fit between a client's decision and skill level; and lastly the difficulties that arise in modifying a client's environment. These junctures in no way represent a comprehensive and exhaustive review of the possible threats to maintaining a client-centred focus, but rather represent an attempt to identify and reflect on some of the everyday issues that affect occupational therapists in mental health settings. At times, the therapists involved identified the need to be directive and override some of the approaches espoused by a client-centred approach. Although this brief abandonment from a client-centred framework is inevitable in mental health settings, the management of this departure represents one of the most significant challenges in client-centred practice.

ACKNOWLEDGEMENTS

The authors thank the following occupational therapists, Claudia Bali, Carrie Clark, Joan Lewis, Edward McAnanama, Susan Nagle, Wendy Parkinson and Anne Wilcox, for their work in submitting the case examples. Their hard work and clinical expertise brought to life many of the issues reviewed in this chapter.

REFERENCES

American Occupational Therapy Association 1993 Core values and attitudes of occupational therapy practice. American Journal of Occupational Therapy 47:1085–1086

Blain J, Townsend E 1993 Occupational therapy guidelines for client-centred practice: impact study findings. Canadian Journal of Occupational Therapy 60(5):271–285

Bruce M A, Christiansen C H 1988 Advocacy in word as well as deed. American Journal of Occupational Therapy 42(3):189–191

Burnard P 1995 Implications of client-centred counselling for nursing practice. Nursing Times 91(26):35–37

Canadian Association of Occupational Therapists 1993 Occupational therapy guidelines for client-centred mental health practice. CAOT Publications ACE, Toronto

Canadian Association of Occupational Therapists 1997 Enabling occupation: an occupational therapy perspective. CAOT Publications ACE, Toronto

Clemens E, Wetle T, Feltes M, Crabtree B, Dubitzky D 1994 Contradictions in case management. Journal of Aging and Health 6(1):70–88

Department of National Health and Welfare, Canadian Association of Occupational Therapists 1983 Guidelines for the client-centred practice of occupational therapy. CAOT Publications ACE, Toronto

Devereaux E B 1984 Occupational therapy's challenge: the caring relationship. American Journal of Occupational Therapy 38(12):791–798

Everett B, Nelson A 1992 We're not cases and you're not managers: an account of a client–professional partnership developed in response to the 'borderline' diagnosis. Psychosocial Rehabilitation Journal 15(4):50–60

Haiman S 1995 Dilemmas in professional collaboration with consumers. Psychiatric Services 46(5):443–445

Krupa T, Clark C C 1995 Occupational therapists as case managers: responding to current approaches to community health service delivery. Canadian Journal of Occupational Therapy 62(1):16–22

Nikkel R E, Smith G, Edwards D 1992 A consumer-operated case management project. Hospital and Community Psychiatry 43:577–579

Paulson R I 1991 Professional training for consumers and family members. Psychosocial Rehabilitation Journal 14:69–80

Peloquin S M 1990 The patient–therapist relationship in occupational therapy: understanding visions and images. American Journal of Occupational Therapy 44(1):13–21

Peloquin S M 1995 The fullness of empathy: reflections and illustrations. American Journal of Occupational Therapy 49(1):24–31

Rosa S A, Hasselkus B R 1996 Connecting with patients: the personal experience of professional helping. Occupational Therapy Journal of Research 16(4):245–260

Rothman J, Smith W, Nakashima J, Paterson M A, Mustin J 1996 Client self-determination and professional intervention: striking a balance. Social Work 41(4):396–405

Wilshaw G 1997 Integration of therapeutic approaches: a new direction for mental health nurses? Journal of Advanced Nursing 26:15–19

Yerxa E J 1994 Dreams, dilemmas, and decisions for occupational therapy practice in a new millennium: an American perspective. American Journal of Occupational Therapy 48(7):586–589

9

Physical disabilities: meeting the challenges of client-centred practice

M. Gage

The issues that arise when interacting with clients who have physical disabilities differ from those in other health settings. This chapter outlines the process of building a solid foundation on which to base a synergistic relationship with the client, and describes how the Interactive Planning Process can be used to determine realistic goals based on client-desired outcomes.

INTRODUCTION

Client-centred practice with clients who have physical health challenges is not inherently different from client-centred practice with any other type of health challenge. Instead it is the issues that arise when interacting with clients who have physical disabilities that are different. This chapter outlines the use of a particular approach, the Interactive Planning Process (M. Gage, unpublished work, 1995). The same process can be applied to clients with many other types of problems. However, the unique issues that arise when applying the process to other disabilities are not addressed in this chapter.

SEVEN DIMENSIONS OF CARE

It is important first to reflect on and develop an understanding of the nature of a client-centred relationship and to evaluate your current practice methods against this measuring stick. The term client centred is sufficiently vague that it can be interpreted differently by different people. Hence, it is important to be aware that your peers and your clients may be using the same term but with different meanings and expectations.

Researchers at the Picker Institute in Boston investigated the experiences of medical and surgical clients and identified the following seven dimensions as key ingredients to a client-centred experience from the perspective of the client (Gerteis et al 1993):

- respect for clients' values, preferences and expressed needs
- coordination and integration of care
- information, communication and education
- physical comfort
- emotional support and alleviation of fear and anxiety
- involvement of family and friends
- transition and continuity.

These seven themes were identified by surveying clients at hospitals across the United States. The themes have since been validated in studies in Canada and the UK (Bruster et al 1994, Charles et al 1994). Hence, regardless of the health system in which you are working, it appears that attention to these seven dimensions of care is critical, from the perspective of clients with physical health problems, to experiencing client-centred care. It is beyond the scope of this chapter to deal with each of these themes in detail. However, it is recommended that individual therapists review the work of Gerteis et al (1993) to determine the degree to which their current practice is client centred from the perspective of the client. The Interactive Planning Process, which will be presented later in this chapter, was designed with the express intention of maximising the client-centred experience by attending to the seven dimensions of care.

THE SYNERGISTIC RELATIONSHIP

The power imbalance between the client and the therapist, as discussed in Chapter 4, creates a barrier to full client participation in any planning process. Power comes from knowledge, social position and/or charisma. When one party has knowledge, social position and/or charisma, that is not equivalent to that held by the other party, the resultant imbalance of power affects the less powerful individual's ability to participate openly in joint decision-making. For this reason, true client-centred practice can occur only when this barrier to the equality of the participants is addressed.

To address this issue it is important to send a message to the client that the knowledge the client has about his or her life and personal illness experience is as valuable to the therapist as the therapist's knowledge of rehabilitation is to the client. The client must perceive that the therapist wishes to develop a synergistic relationship. A synergistic relationship creates a better outcome when the efforts of all participants are combined than could have been created by any one of the participants alone. Compromise is not condoned as an acceptable outcome in that compromise necessitates that both participants sacrifice part of what they wanted in order to find an agreeable solution. Instead, participants in synergistic relationships strive to find synergistic solutions that meet the needs of all participants. The development of a synergistic relationship between the client and the therapist is a key element of all stages of the Interactive Planning Process.

Clients with newly acquired physical disabilities may initially find it difficult to engage in a synergistic relationship. The client may not, yet, have sufficient experience with his or her altered state of abilities to feel competent in participating fully in decision-making related to the condition or to have a sense of what a good outcome might be. At this stage attention must be paid to building a solid foundation upon which the synergistic relationship can grow. This necessitates the development of a common vision that includes hopeful client-desired outcomes; effort is needed by both participants to nurture the relationship on an ongoing basis (Gage 1997). Gage identified 12 subthemes related to building synergistic relationships between all members of the health-care team. This chapter will now examine each of the 12 identified subthemes as they apply to the relationship between a therapist and client who has a physical health challenge.

Building a solid foundation

According to Gage (1997) the process of building a solid foundation upon which to base a synergistic relationship involves:

- Seeing the client as a whole, including
  —acknowledging the strengths along with the problems
  —recognising the impact of the illness on the whole family
  —being willing to assist the client in finding help for issues that are not directly related to the reason for your involvement
  —recognising that the client lives with the disease 24 hours a day and is therefore the expert with respect to his or her illness experience and symptoms.
- The client feeling heard. This involves
  —deep empathic listening that focuses on understanding the other person's experience
  —demonstrating that you have heard
  —changing your actions to be consistent with the new information
  —accepting and attending to issues raised by the client and significant others in the client's life
  —validating concerns, feelings and symptoms
  —accepting expressed desires that are inconsistent with your advice or position
  —believing what you hear from the client.
- Getting to know each other as people, including
  —knowing the client as a person, not just the disease
  —being willing to divulge appropriate personal information to the client.
- Mutual trust in competence, including
  —instilling a sense of competence without misrepresenting or unduly raising hopes of the client
  —health professionals demonstrating a belief in the ability of clients to use their own strengths to rectify problems or issues themselves.
- Establishing a listening environment, including
  —creating a sense that even as a busy therapist you have time to listen to the concerns of your clients

  —finding creative ways to decrease the interruptions when speaking with a client about issues that are meaningful to the client.
- Fostering innovation, including
  —finding ways to create an environment in which the client feels safe enough to shape ideas expressed by the professional or to express ideas that may be contrary to the ideas expressed by the professional
  —avoiding behaviours that limit the possible outcome of the interaction to what the professional believes is realistic.

Establishing a common vision

The setting of goals has been found to be the single most effective means of ensuring that an outcome is attained (Locke & Latham 1990). When a goal stretches you to achieve something that is not a current reality, creative tension emerges. The energy of everyone committed to this goal is directed toward resolving this tension by achieving the outcome. Creative solutions emerge that would not otherwise have been found as the participants work to find a way to resolve the discrepancy between the current reality and the desired future state.

For this reason establishing a common understanding of the desired outcome of the treatment is essential to gaining excellent therapeutic outcomes. When the client has a different expectation with respect to the goal of treatment to the therapist, instead of working together to find creative solutions, there will be conflict that will decrease the chance of success. The conflict will not always be expressed in a direct manner and may manifest itself in a lack of compliance with the instructions of the therapist.

When compliance becomes an issue, it is important that the therapist does not label the client as non-compliant. Such labels serve only to pit the therapist and the client against one another in a power struggle. Instead, the therapist should assume that something is wrong with the plan and endeavour to find out what alternative strategy will work. It may be that the client cannot see the connection between the plan and his or her desired outcome, or that the actions expected of the client cannot occur because of other life commitments that are too pressing to ignore. Explore how the context of the client's life may result in a need to alter the plan. For example, if a client is involved in a law suit related to the course of the disability, he or she may subconsciously, or perhaps even consciously, be afraid that being seen performing some of the actions outlined in the treatment plan may jeopardise the case. If the client is also afraid of never being able to return to work, even if improvement occurs as a result of the therapy, the settlement may be seen as the only way of continuing to support his or her family. As long as the client's desired outcome is to be seen as totally disabled and the therapist's desired outcome is to gain a realistic understanding of the degree of disability, progress will be hampered. A therapist who works through these issues with the client openly and honestly, rather than labelling the client non-compliant, may be able to help the client understand that it is important to be seen as someone who wants to get well.

There may also be a need to develop a documentation process that itemises the activities the client is performing because it is an expectation of the therapeutic process and the client's response to the activity (i.e. pain level during the activity, fatigue after the activity, etc.). Clients involved in legal cases know that they may be secretly videotaped. If the videotaped activities appear to be inconsistent with the degree of disability being claimed, they may negatively affect the outcome of the law suit. The knowledge that this evidence will be seen in context along with a log of the amount of time spent performing the activity, and resultant pain levels, may be sufficient to allay the client's concerns and enable you to develop a common vision for the outcome of treatment.

The establishment of *hopeful* desired outcomes is also an important concept to consider when working with clients with physical disabilities. Health professionals have been trained to be objective in their evaluation of the client's condition and prognosis. The objective evaluations are often based on the average outcome of clients with similar disabilities. However, it is important

that health professionals recognise that some clients defy the odds and achieve what is thought to be impossible (Siegel 1993, Sherr Klein 1997). Clients want to be permitted to maintain their hope for a miracle or, at the very least, a better than average outcome even when all evidence points to the situation being futile. A poignant example of this is related by Gage (1997, p. 180) as she reports on the experience of Patti, a woman who was dying of cancer:

She [Patti] approached an expert on visualization for assistance but was refused help because she expressed a desire to use the visualization techniques to cure her cancer. Her vision of the future was different than the vision of the future the professional was prepared to allow. The visualization expert was prepared to help her only if she would first admit that she was going to die and that the techniques would only increase her comfort during the dying process ... there was an emphasis on making the client accept reality, even when doing so removed the purpose for living. This professional denied [Patti] access to a technique that may have improved her comfort because he believed it was not appropriate for her to hope for a miracle. As health professionals we need to open our minds to work alongside our clients toward hopeful visions of the future.

For the therapist, it may appear to be a waste of precious time to work with a client toward the achievement of an outcome that is highly unlikely to occur. The therapist may need to make choices about the quantity of help each client receives in order to comply with the budgetary restrictions of the employing agency and may be unable to justify working on hopeful outcomes. In addition, if the therapist believes the outcome being sought by the client is unattainable he or she will not be motivated to spend valuable time and resources attempting to gain that outcome (Craig & Craig 1974). However, it is usually possible, after understanding a client's hopeful vision for the future, to break down the steps toward the vision and begin work on a step that is acceptable and believed to be attainable by both the therapist and the client. The therapist should be honest with the client about the chances of attaining the hopeful outcome, while at the same time making a commitment to work with the client toward the hopeful outcome, one attainable step at a time. As the client gains experience with what is possible for him or her, given the onset of a physical disability, the client may voluntarily alter the desired outcome.

Health professionals have a tendency to try to 'fast forward' this adjustment process. By allowing the recognition to occur gradually, the therapist gives the client time to find an acceptable alternative outcome for which to hope before giving up on the more desirable end-result.

Patti's therapist was right to avoid giving Patti the impression that visualisation strategies were likely to cure her cancer. However, instead of insisting that Patti admit that she was going to die before he would agree to teach her visualisation techniques, the therapist could have agreed to help her learn visualisation techniques that would help her improve her comfort. This would have been an interim goal they could both be motivated to work toward.

The ongoing relationship

Synergistic relationships need to be nurtured if they are to be maintained or, even more so, when they are still developing. The following themes were identified by Gage (1997) as being important to this nurturing process: the human touch, reciprocity, feeling valued and having fun.

The human touch

The human touch includes:

- the client's need to be perceived as a human being rather than the object upon which a therapist exerts her professional skills
- the need for the therapist to show that he or she truly cares about what happens to the client as opposed to the process of treatment being simply a job
- the need to spend time with the client exploring issues that are of importance to the client
- the therapist understanding when clients should be encouraged to stretch themselves rather than immediately accepting 'no' for an answer, while at the same time respecting clients' right to self-determination

- the need for the therapist to accomplish all of the above without violating professional boundaries.

Reciprocity

Power can be neutralised in the professional relationship only when both the client and the therapist feel their contribution to the outcome is of equal importance. A sense that both parties are getting and giving something that is essential to the outcome is a key factor. When this is not possible, it is important for the client to be allowed to 'pay back the debt' in other ways. This need is often illustrated in the giving of chocolates or flowers to the therapist. Discretion, on the part of the therapist, is required with respect to the value of the gift that is considered acceptable. When the sense of indebtedness is significant, it may be more appropriate to offer the client the opportunity to contribute to a foundation that will help provide resources for other clients with similar challenges rather than providing a gift that is of direct benefit to the therapist.

Feeling valued

It is not enough to listen to the opinions of clients. It is essential that the opinions be valued and acted upon. When it is impossible to act on the client's opinions because they are contrary to good clinical practice or in some way unethical, it is essential that the rationale for choosing an alternate strategy is discussed fully with the client. There will be times when this discussion does not result in client satisfaction, but at least the client will know that the therapist was not simply ignoring the input.

Having fun

The creation of an environment that is conducive to having fun while working toward desired outcomes is considered important by clients. Clients often find the therapeutic process to be long and difficult. When an element of fun is added, it helps to keep the client motivated. When creating a fun environment emphasis should be placed on creating fun that is respectful of the cultural diversity of the population. People's sense of humour varies and fun that is offensive to a given individual will not create synergy, it will create divisiveness. Given that humour is unique to the individual, every effort should be made to encourage clients to speak up immediately if they are offended by comments. It is also critical that clients do not perceive that you are making light of the seriousness of the challenges being faced.

THE INTERACTIVE PLANNING PROCESS

The Interactive Planning Process was developed with the intention of maximising the client-centred experience with respect to the seven dimensions of care identified by Gerteis et al (1993). This planning process melds together the knowledge, skills and abilities of the client and the therapist in an effort to create the best possible health outcome. The Interactive Planning Process works best when the therapist also attends to the principles of creating a synergistic relationship, as discussed above. The steps of the Interactive Planning Process are reported below as if they occur in a linear fashion. It is important to emphasise that they are in fact each part of an iterative process, with each step being revisited as often as necessary to ensure that new data are integrated into the plan.

Understanding client concerns and expectations

The first step in the process is to gain an in-depth understanding of the client's concerns and/or expectations. This step is a critical foundation piece. Misunderstandings that occur at this stage may create unseen barriers throughout the treatment process. It is important to explore all of the issues outlined in Table 9.1.

The first time you meet a client it will be impossible to gain full disclosure on all the issues outlined in Table 9.1. A complete understanding of all issues will only emerge over the course of time as the client understands that the

therapist values his or her input and finds the information shared to be critical to the treatment process. However, it is important that the therapist attempt to gain a beginning level of understanding of these issues before beginning any other part of the assessment process. Once the therapist has demonstrated his or her knowledge through the assessment and treatment process, the power imbalance will increase, thereby making disclosure even less likely. By seeking information from clients before beginning the 'hands on' assessment process the therapist sends a message to the client that the information clients possess about their illness experience is critical to the process of assessment and treatment. In this way clients begin to believe that they also have power related to the knowledge they possess about their illness experience and the context of their life.

Clinician skills and knowledge

Given that each individual client has a unique illness experience, different knowledge and skills may be required to address the issues and concerns raised by two clients with the same diagnosis. Once the therapist understands the client's perspective, the therapist should reflect on personal skills and abilities to determine whether they are appropriate to address the issues identified. Mutual trust in competence was one of the synergy themes. This trust cannot develop if therapists are afraid to admit to limitations with respect to their skills.

When an issue is identified that falls outside the therapist's skill set, there are several possible choices of action. The therapist may deem the deficit to be so significant that it would be inappropriate to attempt to treat the client. In these circumstances the therapist should discuss alternate sources of help with the client and assist the client in seeking help from the chosen source. The therapist may then go on to address issues that are within his or her skill set. Alternatively, the therapist may be able to acquire the skill required to meet the client's need, even though the issue is one for which the therapist does not currently have expertise. In these circumstances

Table 9.1 The Enabling Interview

Area of exploration	Explanation
Explore how this hospitalisation or health incident has affected the client's life, family, ability to work, etc. General exploration of the meaning of the client's illness to him or her.	This ensures that the health professional is not making any assumptions about the meaning of the illness to the individual that may be based on the 'average' illness experience rather than the actual experience of this client. Gaining this knowledge will help to ensure that priority issues are set in concert with the client's unique illness experience, rather than the average illness experience.
Explore concerns or issues that the client believes are important to address. It is important to explore issues that may be related only indirectly to the health event.	Gaining an understanding of the relative importance of concerns and issues from the perspective of the client will help in the process of setting priorities. It is very important that issues that may indirectly affect decisions are also understood (e.g. wife is also ill and could not be expected to assist with transfers).
Explore the client's desired outcome with respect to the health incident; that is, what does the client wish to see happen.	If the client has a specific outcome that he or she believes will occur before the end of treatment, it is important to know about this at the outset of treatment. In this way the therapist can monitor progress toward this outcome and help the client to readjust expectations if it becomes obvious that the outcome will not be achieved. Many clients do not have well-defined expected outcomes. The role of the therapist is then to assist the client in defining realistic expectations.
Explore any ideas the client has about specific treatments.	If the client begins therapy expecting that a specific treatment is the only thing that will cure him or her and the therapist does not offer that treatment, the client may be resistant to all other treatments. The therapist may label the client as non-compliant when in fact it is a difference in approach that is hampering progress. The therapist may not always be able to offer the desired treatment to the client. The desired treatment may be contraindicated or have been proven to be ineffective. However, it is important to be able to address the reasons for not offering the desired treatment at the outset of the treatment process.
Explore whether the client has any hypotheses about what caused the health event and whether these assumptions are different from those made by the therapist.	For example, if the client believes that the health event is punishment from God for past errors, he or she may not begin to get well until amendment has been made for the past wrongdoings. If the therapist works from the medical model assumption and attempts to rehabilitate only the body, the client may not make gains. Another example is a cardiac client who believes that any exercise will lead to a second attack. It will be impossible to gain the client's cooperation in physical activities until this belief has been challenged successfully.

it is important for the therapist to be open and honest with the client and to discuss with the client the various alternative strategies for seeking help with the issue at hand. It is difficult for a client to refuse help from a professional because of the power differential discussed above. Thus, it is important for the therapist to reassure the client that choosing to seek assistance from an alternative source is an acceptable alternative and will not affect the provision of other services. For example, if you are treating a client who has a fractured hip from an automobile accident and you notice problems with memory, you need to share your concern and recommend an additional evaluation without unnecessarily increasing the client's angst during the process of waiting for the results. Please note that I am not suggesting that information be withheld permanently, only that it be disclosed with sensitivity to the client's situation.

Document client-desired outcomes

The term client-desired outcomes is used to describe the statements that emerge through an interactive process with the client and become the focus of treatment and outcome measurement. Client-desired outcomes are not goals in the usual sense of the word. Generally goals are thought to be realistic, understandable, measurable, behavioural and achievable (Saunders 1984). The client-desired outcome is instead a statement of what the client wants to achieve. It is not limited by what can be measured in objective, behavioural terms. Nor is it limited by the therapist's view of what is realistic. Instead it reflects what the client sees as the desired future state at the time it is written. The client-desired outcome is also not 'carved in stone'. It may change as the client gains more experience with what is possible given the onset of the physical limitations related to the illness or disease. As such, the client-desired outcome is written, as if by the client, in the first person.

The client's perceived self-efficacy, that is the client's perceived ability to perform a specific task, is based on efficacy information that is no longer accurate given the new limitations being experienced (Bandura 1986). As such, the client cannot be expected to have a realistic sense of what is achievable. Nor can the client be expected to become 'realistic' as soon as the therapist explains his or her view of what is realistic. There is instead a need to support the client in experimenting with what is possible, given the new physical limitations. When the client-desired outcome is considered to be unachievable by the therapist, the therapist should first consider whether there is an interim outcome that is realistic and that would lead the client toward the desired outcome – remember the earlier discussion about the importance of allowing the client to set *hopeful* desired outcomes.

Another important issue with respect to the setting of client-desired outcomes is the understanding of how the outcomes are derived. The therapist should avoid the use of the terms 'goal' and 'client-desired outcome'. These concepts are used in this document to assist the clinician in understanding the process of planning. The term goal is a sophisticated four-letter word that must be avoided unless treating a client who understands the concept. In addition, because client's do not have experience with what is possible, given their new physical limitations and lack of health-care experience, the client may wish to rely on the therapist for guidance in setting goals. While clients often do not have an answer to the question 'What is your goal?', they do know what their concerns are and what is important for them to be able to do again.

From the information collected using the Enabling Interview (Table 9.1) the therapist gains an understanding of what issues the client wishes to address and whether the client believes that any specific strategies will be effective in addressing these issues. The therapist also has knowledge of outcomes that have been achieved by similar clients. Through an interactive process which values both the concerns of the client and the clinical knowledge of the therapist, the therapist can help the client to define statements of desired outcomes that reflect the concerns, issues and strategies identified by the client during the Enabling Interview. The therapist must make sure that the meaning of the client's earlier statements are not changed as a result of the clinician's tendency to want to arrive at realistic, measureable, achievable outcome statements.

General hypotheses

Clients state that their individual preferences, values and expressed needs are not being considered when treatment plans are developed (Gerteis et al 1993). Rogers and Holm (1991) note that therapists begin to generate their hypotheses about what is wrong and what treatment may be indicated as soon as they read the diagnosis on the chart. This means that much treatment planning is occurring before there is a true understanding of the client's unique illness experience or desired outcomes.

Once the client-desired outcomes have been developed, it is important to determine whether this new information suggests new hypotheses. Hypotheses are sometimes so firmly entrenched that they are assumed to be true for all clients. For example, an occupational therapist heard the diagnosis spinal cord injury and hypothesised that the injury had impaired the client's ability to dress independently and that regaining independence in dressing would be a desired outcome of the treatment programme. The process of dressing was so exhausting that this particular client chose to hire an attendant to assist him with dressing so that he would have energy left to do the things that were really important in his life. This client had wanted to stop the dressing programme much earlier, but was afraid of hurting the therapist's feelings if he told her his plan. Many weeks of valuable treatment time were wasted attempting to resolve issues related to independent dressing simply because the therapist was working from the wrong hypothesis. Had she taken the time to explore with the client the meaning of various occupations, a different hypotheses may have been used in planning treatment and valuable treatment time would have been saved.

The hypothesis that all clients want to be independent in dressing was so firmly entrenched in this therapist's mind that she did not consider other possible responses of the client. It is also important to note that this client's view of the importance of independence in dressing changed during the course of treatment. It was only when he experienced the exhaustion brought on by attempting to dress independently that he changed his view. This illustrates the importance of remembering that the Interactive Planning Process is an iterative, as opposed to linear, process. Provision must be made to facilitate changes in the desired outcomes of treatment as new information becomes known or, as in this case, the client gains more experience with the consequences of the disability.

Client resources

According to literature on client empowerment it is important to send a strong message to clients that it is within their power to affect the state of their own health (Rappaport 1985). To this end, the next step in the Interactive Planning Process

is for the therapist to help the client identify the potential ways in which he or she can contribute to a successful outcome. The client's role should not be expressed as 'to cooperate with the treatment process'. This still leaves the client in a somewhat passive role with respect to taking control of the future. In addition, it does not lay out a specific course of action that is required of the client. Instead the possible contribution would be stated specifically. For example: 'to do a home programme daily' or 'to call suppliers to find the most inexpensive adapted bath seat'.

The final statement of client contribution cannot be made until the full assessment has been completed and the initial treatment plan finalised. The purpose of starting to identify such contributions early is to promote a sense that the client has a role to play if a good outcome is to be achieved. By looking for clients' strengths, rather than concentrating solely on problems, the therapist increases the chance that clients will actively search for solutions themselves rather than passively waiting for the therapist to cure them. The combined efforts of the client and therapist are more likely to result in success than the effort of only one.

It is important to discuss openly the concept of helping oneself improve. For some clients there is an expectation that the therapist has a magic wand to wave that will make them well again. For others, there is a belief that it is inappropriate for health professionals to expect the client to do the health professional's work. It is important to clarify that the individual is responsible for his or her own health and that the role of the professional is to provide the expertise needed to overcome barriers to wellness, as opposed to being wholly responsible for the cure.

Assess barriers

Now that the therapist has a good understanding of what the client is trying to achieve and what contribution the client is prepared to make, it is time to begin the process of identifying what stands in the way of the client's success. The therapist is expected to use all possible professional knowledge and skill in an effort to assist the client in achieving client-desired outcomes and in identifying issues that may be important, but not apparent, to the client.

The assessment should be streamlined to be consistent with the client's desired outcomes. Achieving holistic practice is more a factor of assessing all aspects of client functioning that are related to client-desired outcomes than of assessing and treating all possible problems. Having said that, it is also critical that the assessment encompass components that are essential to the identification of important issues about which the client may have no knowledge.

Being client centred does not mean attending only to issues raised by the client. The therapist is trained to understand issues that may arise within specific diagnostic categories, and thus will have knowledge about issues that must be shared with the client. Ignoring issues because the client does not identify them would not be client centred. However, once the issue has been identified, if it is still unimportant to the client the therapist should be prepared to defer to client choice unless the decision presents a threat to others or the client is not competent to decide. It is important that the therapist make every effort to ensure that the client understands the ramifications of the decision but, ultimately, the therapist must respect the client's choice and avoid using professional power to sway the client's choice. For example, if during the course of an assessment of a client who had a broken leg you became concerned about the presence of a learning disability, you would provide the client with information about your concerns and possible courses of action. The client who has adapted to the disability may not wish to pursue assessment and treatment. Provided the client is considered competent to decide, and given that there is no apparent risk to the client or others, the therapist should respect the right to refuse treatment.

Validate assessment findings

Once the assessment is complete, it is important to share the analysis of the results with the client to provide a new perspective on the assessment data. For example, when assessing a client's ability to return to work the therapist might be looking for maximum voluntary effort indicators. If you identify indicators of inconsistent effort and share these thoughts with the client, you provide the client with an opportunity to disclose any fear of reinjury or of bringing on a second heart attack. This provides an alternative interpretation for the data that may be important to your conclusions.

Negotiate specific treatment goals

Now that the assessment is finalised it is time to develop specific treatment goals that are consistent with the client-desired outcomes. These statements will be specific and measurable indicators of the direction of treatment. If the assessment results uncover issues that change the client-desired outcomes, these should also be modified.

Gain client commitment

Once treatment goals are established, the client should be asked to make a commitment to working toward each goal. The connection between these goals and the client's desired outcome should be articulated specifically so that there is little chance of misunderstanding.

Design and implement a specific action plan

Once the client has committed to the goals, the specific action plan to attain those goals can be developed and implemented.

Evaluate

The appropriate time for evaluation will vary from situation to situation and will be related to the desired outcomes being addressed and the speed with which individual goals are expected to be attained. When it is time to evaluate the outcome it is important to ensure that the evaluation examines whether the client-desired outcomes have been achieved rather than evaluating whether the goals have been achieved. The biggest mistake therapists make is to evaluate the effectiveness of the programme by evaluating the attainment of the goals that were derived in an attempt to achieve the desired outcomes. The attainment of the specific goals becomes inconsequential if their attainment does not in turn bring the client closer to the desired outcomes articulated in the first stage of the process. The goals were defined by breaking down the desired outcome into manageable steps. It may be that there was a fault in the reasoning that led to the selection of a specific goal and, hence, the attainment of that goal may not result in the attainment of the desired outcome.

Evaluation can be performed in one of the following three ways:

- You can use a dichotomous measure of 'yes' or 'no'. In this case you would ask the client: 'Has this outcome been accomplished to your satisfaction?'. The client would answer 'yes' or 'no'. The success of treatment would be dependent upon how many 'yes' responses were achieved. It is appropriate for the client to answer 'yes' to a question when it is about an outcome that has become irrelevant during the course of treatment. It is also acceptable for this outcome simply to be removed from the list, and considered to be accomplished, at the time it becomes irrelevant during treatment. There is no sense continuing to work on outcomes that have been resolved in terms of importance to the client.
- Goal attainment scaling (Kiresuk & Sherman 1968) can be used. It is beyond the scope of this chapter to outline this process fully. Instead the reader is referred to references that specifically address this strategy (Kirshner & Guyatt 1985, Lewis et al 1987, Lloyd 1986, Ottenbacher & Cusick 1993). The strength of goal attainment scaling is the ability to derive a standard score that enables the comparison of groups of clients in terms of their progress. However, the process requires that each goal have five levels of

possible outcome. It is sometimes difficult to develop five levels without changing the meaning of the outcome to the client.
- The measurement scale used for the Canadian Occupational Performance Measure (COPM) (Law et al 1994) is another choice. This scale requires that the client score each desired outcome with respect to its importance, the client's perceived ability to accomplish the item today, and the client's satisfaction with the noted level of perceived ability. The advantage of this scale is that it shows progress toward the desired outcome, rather than indicating only whether it was fully achieved or not. The disadvantage is that it does not indicate whether the degree of improvement was sufficient to make a difference in the client's life, although a change in the satisfaction score certainly connotes increased client satisfaction with performance. A combination of the dichotomous measure and the COPM measure may be advisable. This system is only adaptable to behavioural and performance-related desired outcomes. Outcomes such as 'I want a pain-free insertion of my temporary line' are not able to be rated on this scale. This was a desired outcome for a dialysis client. Most occupational therapy outcomes would be appropriate for the COPM system.

If at the time of evaluation you find that the desired outcomes have been achieved, the client can be discharged from treatment. When you find that the desired outcomes have not been achieved and that progress toward the outcomes is not occurring, it is time to revisit each step of the Interactive Planning Process. There is a tendency to re-examine the specific treatment plan rather than questioning whether perhaps the therapist does not understand the client's concerns or something about the context of the client's life that may be affecting the client's progress. The first steps of the Interactive Planning Process are considered to be foundation pieces and as such, when an error is made in the early stages, it may affect the whole process.

In addition, the process of attempting to treat the client may have led to the discovery of new information that may affect the desired outcomes that are being sought. If one does not make a conscious effort to re-examine each step in the process, the meaning of the new information may not be fully understood.

In addition to measuring outcome according to whether the desired outcomes were achieved, it is important to ensure that other critical outcome factors are also being tracked. For example, if you are working with a client with reduced range of motion, it may be appropriate to monitor range of motion. While improving range of motion may not be one of the expressed client-desired outcomes, a change in range of motion would provide the therapist with valuable information upon which to base changes in treatment. An evaluation that solely used client input is not adequate to ensure that you, as an occupational therapist, provide the best advice and input to the development of an appropriate treatment programme.

SITUATIONS THAT CHALLENGE CLIENT-CENTRED PRACTICE

When goals of the client and family differ

When the desired outcomes of family members are different from those of the competent client, it is important to attempt first to find a synergistic solution that will satisfy the needs of all involved parties. It must be recognised that the family member may be as affected by the choice being made as the client. The client does not live in a vacuum and a client's choice may have significant effects on family members. The client is, in effect, part of a system: when one part of the system changes, effects are felt on other parts of the system. Failure to consider these effects may lead to a poor decision, and a poor outcome. First try to understand the concerns of each participant and what they are attempting to achieve. Next create an environment conducive to brainstorming solutions that will meet all desired outcomes. This process often results in synergistic solutions that resolve the conflict.

It is recognised that all situations cannot be resolved. When it becomes impossible to meet the needs of all participants, the therapist must give priority to the desired outcomes of the client (giving consideration first to any applicable regional laws).

Dealing with moral dilemmas

Therapists encounter situations where the client's desired outcomes conflict with the beliefs of the therapist. For example, the therapist may be asked to provide treatment to enable a client to accomplish a desired outcome that the therapist considers to be unsafe. Provided the client is competent and the outcome is not endangering others, illegal or morally corrupt, the therapist may have an obligation to allow the client to 'live at risk'. Laws regarding such choices are regionally different. Thus, therapists should endeavour to understand the laws governing their practice environment and seek legal counsel when in doubt.

Morally challenging situations require that therapists, in order to protect themselves from litigation, seek advice and support from colleagues. When placed in a situation where they believe they are assisting a client to harm him or herself, there is a need to seek help dealing with the emotional consequences to the therapist.

When the moral dilemma relates to a client wishing to engage in an activity that challenges the therapist's moral standards, the therapist should attempt to find an alternative source of help for the client. For example, a client who wishes assistance with positioning in order to engage in premarital sex may encounter a therapist opposed to premarital sex. It is important that therapists do not attempt to force their moral position on to the client. Instead, the therapist should refer the client to another occupational therapist for whom this moral dilemma does not exist.

When you are part of a team

It is possible for one member of a team to use the Interactive Planning Process to plan his or her aspects of treatment without commitment from all team members. When at least one member of the team is using this process, that team member can advocate for the client perspective within team meetings. It is preferable, when there are multiple team members, that the Interactive Planning Process be used by the whole team. In this way the opinions and skills of all members of the team, including the client as a significant member of the team, are taken into consideration. Gage (1994) presents a strategy for coordinating the work of the team around the desired outcomes identified by the client. Essentially, one member of the team acts as a primary contact with the client to begin the Interactive Planning Process. One set of desired outcomes that are accepted by all team members is developed. Each member of the team then interacts with the

client to determine the unique role of that discipline with respect to attaining the client's desired outcome.

CONCLUSION

Clients with physical disabilities are more likely to experience therapy as client centred when the therapist attends to the 12 subthemes identified with respect to creating a synergistic relationship (Gage 1997) and follows the Interactive Planning Process (M. Gage, unpublished work, 1995). This process integrates the desired outcomes and abilities of the client and the skills and abilities of the therapist. In addition to the client experiencing a client-centred process, the therapist feels gratified by the progress made by the client, to which the therapist has contributed.

REFERENCES

Bandura A 1986 Social foundations of thought and action. Prentice Hall, Englewood Cliffs, New Jersey

Bruster S, Jarman B, Bosanquet N, Weston D, Erens R 1994 National survey of hospital patients. British Medical Journal 309:1542–1546

Charles C, Gauld M, Chambers L, O'Brien B, Haynes R B, Labelle R 1994 How was your hospital stay? Patients' reports about their care in Canadian hospitals. Canadian Medical Association Journal 150(11):1813–1822

Craig J H, Craig M 1974 Synergic power: beyond domination and permissiveness. ProActive Press, Berkeley, California

Gage M 1994 The patient-driven interdisciplinary care plan. Journal of Nursing Administration 24(4):26–35

Gage M 1997 From independence to interdependence: creating synergistic health care teams. Canadian Journal of Occupational Therapy 64:174–183

Gerteis M, Edgman-Levitan S, Daley J, Delbanco T 1993 Through the patient's eyes. Jossey-Bass, San Francisco

Kiresuk T, Sherman R 1968 Goal attainment scaling: a general method of evaluating comprehensive mental health programs. Community Mental Health Journal 4:443–453

Kirshner B, Guyatt G 1985 A methodologic framework for assessing health indices. Journal of Chronic Diseases 38:27–36

Law M, Baptiste S, Carswell A, McColl M A, Polatajko H, Pollock N 1994 Canadian occupational performance measure, 2nd edn. CAOT Publications ACE, Ottawa

Lewis A B, Spencer J H, Haas G L, DiVittis A 1987 Goal attainment scaling: relevance and replicability in follow-up of inpatients. Journal of Nervous and Mental Disorders 175:408–417

Lloyd C 1986 The process of goal setting using goal attainment scaling in a therapeutic community. Occupational Therapy in Mental Health 6(3):19–30

Locke E, Latham G 1990 A theory of goal setting and task performance. Prentice Hall, Englewood Cliffs, New Jersey

Ottenbacher K, Cusick A 1993 Discriminative versus evaluative assessment: some observations on goal attainment scaling. American Journal of Occupational Therapy 47:349–354

Rappaport J 1985 The power of empowerment language. Social Policy 16:15–21

Rogers J C, Holm M B 1991 Occupational therapy diagnostic reasoning: a component of clinical reasoning. American Journal of Occupational Therapy 45(11):1045–1053

Saunders B 1984 Muriel Driver Memorial Lecture 1984 Quality assurance – reflection on the wave. Canadian Journal of Occupational Therapy 51:161–170

Sherr Klein B 1997 Slow dance: a story of stroke, love and disability. Vintage Canada, Toronto

Siegel B 1993 How to live between office visits. Harper Collins, New York

10

The Canadian Occupational Performance Measure

N. Pollock
M. A. McColl
A. Carswell

This chapter describes the Canadian Occupational Performance Measure (COPM), an outcome measure based on the Canadian Model of Occupational Performance and the Occupational Therapy Guidelines for Client-centred Practice. The COPM and its development are described; evidence of reliability, validity, utility and responsiveness are presented; the challenges in using the COPM are discussed and some case examples presented to illustrate its use in practice.

This chapter describes the Canadian Occupational Performance Measure (COPM), an individualised outcome measure designed for use by occupational therapists within a client-centred practice. An overview of outcome measurement is presented followed by a description of the COPM and the process of its development. The psychometric properties are described followed by a discussion of the challenges inherent in using the COPM. The chapter concludes with three case scenarios as examples of the use of the COPM.

OUTCOME MEASUREMENT

In the health-care delivery system, standardised measures from which inferences can be drawn about the quality of care are essential to support professional practice. Donabedian (1976) has classified three assessment approaches to gathering information about the effectiveness of therapy: structure (the attributes of the settings in which interventions are provided), process (what is actually done during intervention) and outcome (the effects of intervention on the disability of the client). There is a reciprocal relationship among these three assessment approaches; good structure increases the likelihood of a good process, and good process increases the likelihood of a good outcome. It is a good idea to include all elements of structure, process and outcome when examining intervention programmes (Donabedian 1993). For the purposes of this chapter, the focus will be on outcome measures.

Traditionally outcome measures have been adverse events such as mortality or morbidity statistics which often focused upon institutional care processes. More recently the trend has been to measure outcomes across the continuum of care and not just at the end of the process. Therefore, alternative outcome measures include quality of life measures, health status measures, changes in clients' health status, changes in clients' knowledge about their disability or behaviours, and the degree of clients' satisfaction with the intervention they receive.

In occupational therapy, outcome measures determine the effects of occupational therapy interventions on clients' occupational performance. They should define the occupational performance consequences of the therapeutic actions which are the product of equal and fully informed participation of clients and therapists. Specifically occupational therapy outcome measures are systematic methods to determine the qualitative and quantitative impacts of an intervention or a programme of interventions. They include measures that are standardised, reliable, valid and that are sensitive to change, which allow therapists to attribute client performance outcomes to the interventions they have provided.

How is an outcome measure selected?

The goal of occupational therapy outcome measurement is to provide an empirical basis for clinical decision-making (Ellenberg 1996, Higgins 1997). However, there a number of issues that must be addressed when selecting an outcome measure. In addition to the usual psychometric attributes of reliability, validity and

responsiveness, there must be a framework or a model of occupational therapy practice which enables the therapist and the client to determine and agree upon the attributes to be measured. The timing of the assessments must be determined, and the reasons for assessing outcome should be defined. Then the issue of attribution can be addressed.

A model or framework for occupational therapy practice permits therapists and clients to define the objectives or goals of intervention, the means of intervention and the desired performance outcomes. Once the desired outcomes have been generated, an outcome measure can be selected. Timing is another important consideration. When is outcome measured? At the completion of the intervention, part way through or at negotiated points throughout the intervention process? Repeated measures of outcome over time allow stronger inferences to be made regarding the effectiveness of the intervention. The reason for assessing outcomes impinges upon the selection of a measure. Different reasons require different types of outcome measures. A measure that is used to determine the effect of a specific intervention will be different from one used to determine the effects of a programme, or for the purpose of improving the quality of care.

The final aspect of attribution is the most difficult to address. The question is, can the attribution of occupational therapy 'cause and effect' be determined in an interdisciplinary programme? When therapists have selected an outcome measure based on a clearly identified model of practice and desired occupational performance outcomes, when there are repeated measures, when the selected instrument demonstrates empirical evidence of reliability, validity and responsiveness, and measures the performance attribute, then attribution is justified.

Individualised outcome measurement

Rogers & Holm (1994) noted that clients who receive occupational therapy services have specific expectations from the service. They have the right to expect that the therapist selects an appropriate intervention based on empirical evidence and which is effective; that the intervention is appropriate to their unique therapeutic needs; and that the intervention is consistent with their stated goals. These expectations reflect an implicit contract between the occupational therapist and the client, and they need to be measured in some manner.

The most useful instrument for measuring the effectiveness of this contract is an individualised outcome measurement. An individualised outcome measure is one that reflects the change in the performance aspirations and satisfaction of the client, demonstrates the effectiveness of the occupational therapy intervention, and is psychometrically robust. It can be used to inform and engage the client in the therapeutic process, yet is sufficient to provide useful data to examine treatment efficacy. The Canadian Occupational Performance Measure (COPM) is one such measure.

DESCRIPTION OF THE COPM

The COPM is an individualised measure in the form of a semistructured interview designed to measure a client's self-perception of occupational performance. It was developed for use by occupational therapists and, as such, focuses on occupational performance. The COPM can be used as a screening tool to determine whether the client requires the services of an occupational therapist; in an initial assessment to help the therapist and client understand the nature of the occupational performance problems an individual is experiencing and assist in setting the goals for therapy; and as an outcome measure to determine the degree of change in occupational performance the client experiences over time as a result of intervention. The COPM can be administered to an individual client, to others in the client's environment (e.g. family, caregiver, teacher), or may be used in situations where the client is not an individual, but rather an organisation, such as a nursing home or factory. The COPM is not age or diagnosis specific, so can be used with a wide variety of clients.

The COPM is based on the *Occupational therapy guidelines for client-centred practice* (CAOT 1991) and the Canadian Model of Occupational Performance (CAOT 1991, 1997). The COPM is a tool that operationalises the main concepts in these models. The focus is on occupational performance areas, namely self-care, productivity and leisure. The client's perspective is sought through the interview process, and occupational performance problems are defined by the client. The COPM incorporates the client's roles and role expectations, and considers the individual's environment, thereby ensuring that the issues identified are relevant for the client.

The occupational performance process (Fig. 10.1) describes the steps through which clients and therapists proceed in occupational therapy (CAOT 1997). The first step is to name, validate and prioritise the occupational performance problems. This is the step where the COPM can be used initially. It allows the client to express the areas of concern in daily occupational performance and to indicate the priority of those concerns. From there, the therapist selects a theoretical perspective and moves to a second level of assessment, seeking to understand why the client is experiencing the problems identified. These steps include assessing performance components, examining the environment, and identifying strengths and resources within the client or the client's situation. The COPM is not designed to be used in these steps. It is targeted at understanding the presenting occupational performance problems from the client's perspective. There are many other tools and methods available to assist in the completion of steps 3 and 4 of the occupational performance process.

Once a plan has been formulated and implemented (steps 5 and 6), the final step is to evaluate outcomes. Again, this is where the COPM can be used. Clients can score their performance and satisfaction with performance in the areas identified through the COPM completed in step 1. The COPM can be used at the beginning and at the end of the occupational performance process.

The COPM is a standardised instrument, in that there are specific instructions and methods for administering and scoring the test; however,

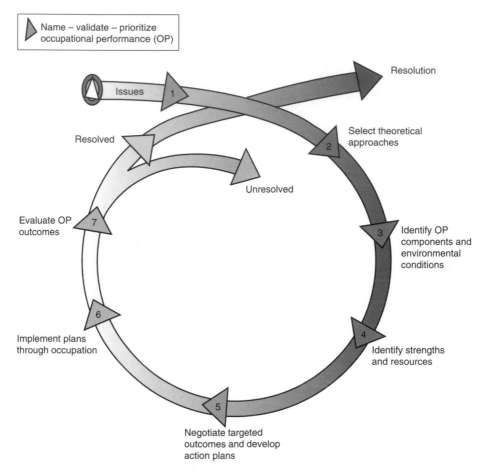

Figure 10.1 Model of the occupational performance process. (Reproduced with kind permission of CAOT Publications from Fearing V, Law M, Clark J 1997 An occupational performance process model: fostering client and therapist alliances. Canadian Journal of Occupational Therapy 64(1):7–15)

it is not a norm-referenced measure. It was not designed to assess deviations in occupational performance from some empirically driven norm. In fact, no such norm exists and, even if one did, it would be inconsistent with the theoretical basis of the COPM to apply a population-based standard to occupational performance. The theoretical base upon which the measure was developed describes occupational performance as an individual, subjective experience.

DEVELOPMENT OF THE COPM

During the 1980s, a series of task forces began to articulate a philosophy of practice for Canadian occupational therapists. These projects resulted

in a series of publications describing a client-centred approach to the practice of occupational therapy (Department of National Health and Welfare (DNHW) & CAOT 1983, 1986, 1987). The third publication investigated the area of outcome measurement in occupational therapy and made the recommendation that 'a tool or set of tools ... be developed ... specifically for occupational therapy' (DNHW & CAOT 1987). The COPM was developed in response to this recommendation. A critical review of the outcome measures used by occupational therapists revealed a number of shortcomings (Pollock et al 1990). Of the 136 measures evaluated, only 54 measured some aspect of occupational performance. Other limitations included a lack of involvement of the client in the process and little emphasis on role expectations or the impact of the client's environment. There did not appear to be an existing measure that met the criteria set out by the task force, and so the COPM was developed.

PSYCHOMETRIC PROPERTIES OF THE COPM

The initial development and pilot testing of the measure were completed in several phases and involved occupational therapists and clients from 55 test sites in Canada, Britain, New Zealand and Greece (Law et al 1994a). Since that time, a number of studies have been conducted by the authors and by other investigators to determine the utility, reliability, responsiveness and validity of the COPM.

Utility

The results from several studies show that the majority of COPM users found it is easy to administer. The typical time to complete the COPM was 30–45 minutes (Law et al 1994b, McColl et al 1997, Toomey et al 1995). The time taken to administer the COPM is influenced by whether the therapist and client stick to assessment; if they begin to analyse and solve the problems identified, then the administration time is lengthened. Therapists commented that the COPM provided a useful framework for their initial assessment and helped them to implement a client-centred approach. Some therapists have also found the COPM helps to clarify the role of the occupational therapist for the client and for other members of the health-care team (Law et al 1994b, Toomey et al 1995).

From the client's perspective, most found that the COPM helped them to define their occupational problems more clearly, to consider their personal priorities, and to understand the role of occupational therapy. Some clients were not used to identifying their own problems for intervention and found the process overwhelming. Others had difficulty shifting their expectations from therapist as expert to client as expert.

For some, however, this was very empowering and they enjoyed the opportunity to become a partner in their own rehabilitation.

Reliability

In an outcome measure, it is particularly important to establish the stability of the measure over time, so you can have confidence that changes seen in scores on reassessment are due to changes in the client, not error in the measure. Four studies have examined the test–retest reliability of the COPM (Bosch 1995, Law et al 1994a, Sanford et al 1994, M. Law & D. Stewart, personal communication, 1996). The study samples included a variety of clients of differing ages and disabilities and COPMs administered in various service settings (e.g. community, institutional). Intraclass correlation coefficients ranged from 0.63 to 0.80 for the Performance scores and from 0.75 to 0.89 for the Satisfaction scores, indicating acceptable to high reliability.

Responsiveness

Responsiveness refers to the ability of the COPM to detect change over time. Responsiveness was evaluated as part of the pilot study, and results showed significant differences between initial and reassessment scores for both Performance and Satisfaction scores ($P < 0.0001$, df = 138). Sanford et al (1994) also found significant COPM score changes following a 3-month outpatient day programme for seniors ($P < 0.001$). In this same study, changes in overall function as perceived by caregivers, therapists and clients were compared to COPM scores and found to have moderate levels of correlation. Law and colleagues (1991), in a study investigating the effects of neurodevelopmental therapy and upper extremity casting on hand function, compared COPM change scores to global change scores and found a moderate correlation.

Validity

Content validity of the COPM is supported by the process through which it was developed

(Bosch 1995). As well, the COPM has come to represent a standard for measurement in research, practice and education in occupational therapy as evidenced by the conference presentations, citations and translations into other languages (Baptiste et al 1993, Steeden 1994, Trombly 1993).

Criterion validity has been assessed by comparing COPM scores with scores achieved on measures of the same construct. McColl et al (1997) compared problems identified on the COPM with those identified spontaneously in response to the question: 'What are the five most important problems that you experience in daily living?'. Results showed the respondents identified similar problems, although the structured approach of the COPM tended to elicit more problems. Pollock & Stewart (1998) had similar findings when using the COPM with teachers, parents and children with disabilities. The COPM was compared with an open-ended interview. The COPM was more successful in identifying problems of individual occupational performance, whereas the open-ended question was more inclined to raise issues at the family, school or broader system level. There was an average congruence between the two methods of three of five problems identified.

Bosch (1995) offered evidence of criterion validity through moderate relationships between the COPM and other well-known measures including the Medical Outcomes Study 36-item short-form health survey (SF-36) (Ware & Sherbourne 1992) and the Structured Assessment of Independent Living Skills (SAILS) (Mahurin et al 1991). The SF-36 is a health status measure which assesses several domains, including physical function, social and role function, mental health, energy/fatigue, pain and general health. SAILS measures activities of daily living and instrumental activities of daily living, and categorises function into cognitive and motor tasks.

McColl and colleagues (1997) provided evidence for construct validity in a recent study. The theory base in occupational therapy asserts that occupational performance is intrinsically satisfying (Yerxa et al 1988); that it is an integral aspect of independent living (Trombly 1993); and that it

is inherently related to life satisfaction (Meyer 1922, Slagle 1934). Thus measures of occupational performance should, theoretically, show some relationship with these other constructs. McColl and colleagues (1997), using both univariate and multivariate methods (and controlling for age, sex and severity of disability), showed a high degree of correlation between COPM scores and scores on measures of each of these three theoretically related constructs. COPM Performance scores were related to scores on the Reintegration to Normal Living Index (Wood-Dauphinee et al 1988) and the Life Satisfaction Scale (Michalos 1985). COPM Satisfaction scores were related to scores on the Satisfaction with Performance Scaled Questionnaire (Yerxa et al 1988) and the Life Satisfaction Scale.

In summary, the evidence available to date indicates that the COPM is a clinically useful measure, having adequate to high test–retest reliability, significant responsiveness, and good content, criterion and construct validity.

CHALLENGES IN USING THE COPM

Many occupational therapists choose to use the COPM as part of the initial assessment process. As this initial assessment is often the first contact between therapist and client, it takes on tremendous importance in establishing the nature of the relationship. In a client-centred approach, therapists must make it clear to clients that they are interested in the client's view of the situation, that they want to understand the context of the client's situation, that the therapist has some relevant expertise to offer, and that client and therapist will be working in partnership throughout the therapy process. The COPM can be a useful tool to communicate these concepts. The domain of concern of the COPM, occupational performance, clearly articulates to clients that, as occupational therapists, we are interested in the client's daily occupations. We want to understand the occupations in which the clients are typically engaged and any problems the client is experiencing. Through the scoring of the COPM, we show that we are interested in clients' perception of their own performance and satisfaction with that performance, and want clients to determine where the priorities lie for the therapy process. The COPM provides a structure that allows the client to communicate these ideas clearly to the therapist, as well as providing a baseline measure which can later be used to evaluate change. As stated earlier, the COPM allows occupational therapists to operationalise the beliefs and assumptions of client-centred practice.

Our experience and research with the COPM, as well as some of the work of other investigators, has shown that therapists who are more comfortable practising from a client-centred model are quite comfortable using the COPM, whereas those used to a more professionally driven model have difficulty using the COPM (Pollock & Stewart 1998, Toomey et al 1995). Using the COPM, the client identifies the areas of concern, not the therapist. The role of the therapist is to understand the reasons for the difficulties, and to work with the client to overcome those difficulties; however, it is essential that the client describe the areas of concern. The client holds the expertise in describing the problem. The therapist's expertise lies in the analysis of the reasons for the problem.

Many therapists believe that they routinely ask clients about their perspectives and priorities, there is some evidence that this may not be the case. Neistadt (1995) surveyed occupational therapists working in adult physical rehabilitation facilities across the United States to assess the degree to which therapists incorporated client priorities into their treatment. Of the 267 respondents, 99% reported that they routinely identified client priorities upon admission to therapy. In contrast, Northen et al (1995) found through observation of initial assessments, again in adult physical rehabilitation settings, only 37% of therapists tried to elicit clients' concerns and none of the therapists asked the clients to establish priorities of concern. The gap between self-reported actions and observed actions seems very significant. These studies serve to show the difficulties some therapists are experiencing in trying to operationalise some of the basic principles of client-centred practice.

While the COPM can facilitate a client-centred relationship, this is rarely a simple thing to accomplish. Where a client can clearly articulate his or her occupational performance concerns and priorities, administration of the COPM is easy. However, for the majority of clients seeking occupational therapy services, eliciting a list of priority problems will be more challenging. Clients may have cognitive impairments which limit their insight or ability to understand the COPM. They may speak a different language or have a communication difficulty which limits their ability to respond. They may be experiencing significant emotional turmoil and have difficulty in decision-making or simply be unused to being asked for their opinion in a health-care context.

There are many factors that will increase the difficulty in using the COPM, and place greater challenges on the therapist. It is then incumbent on the therapist who wishes to remain true to a client-centred approach to be creative in gaining the required information. Some clients simply need more time to think about the questions or more time to respond. Some will require the development of a more solid relationship with the therapist first. They may require a higher level of trust to develop before feeling comfortable in responding. For some, the process may need to be made more concrete, for example walking through a typical day's schedule with the client to help them describe areas of occupational performance that are more disrupted or more important to them. Some clients may need more help in understanding the rating scales or more examples of things we typically rate to help them use the scales in a meaningful way.

For some clients, for example young children or those with significant cognitive impairment, the COPM will need to be done with family or caregivers rather than with the clients themselves. Here it is important to emphasise that the respondent is describing his or her own perspective and not answering as a proxy for the individual client. For example, the mother of a young child with cerebral palsy is being asked how important it is to her that the child can learn to dress him or herself, not how important it is for the child. Respondents cannot truly know how someone else feels and, therefore, can really give only their own perspective. It is also important that the therapist initially give the client the benefit of the doubt and try the COPM with the individual. Many therapists have reported being surprised by the level of insight of particular clients whom they anticipated would be unable to respond to the COPM.

There are times when the therapist will question the information received from the client; this is particularly an issue if the therapist considers that the client is at risk. For example, an elderly client living alone may not perceive that she is having any difficulties around the home, but the therapist may believe her to be at high risk for falling. Here the therapist may need to take a more directive approach in pointing out her concerns to the client and working towards a solution. Wherever possible, input from family and/or caregivers may be helpful in resolving these types of dilemmas. Where a client is unconcerned, the family may be very concerned and identify a number of problems. In these circumstances, the therapist will need to engage in some negotiation, or some decision-making, around who is the primary client.

Another area of difficulty that therapists have reported in using the COPM is time. The results of several studies reported earlier indicate the COPM takes an average of 30–45 minutes to administer. Within some health-delivery systems, the therapists have indicated the COPM takes too much time. The COPM definitely requires an investment of time, but, like most investments, one hopes there is a pay-off. If the time is taken to understand the client's perspective initially, therapy goals will be easy to establish and you and the client will be clear about the direction of therapy. The baseline evaluation has been done, and the re-evaluation using the COPM is quick and easy. This ease of reassessment will facilitate examination of progress in a more systematic way and may facilitate earlier discharge from therapy and increased client satisfaction with the process. By having the client identify priorities, the second level of assessment may be shortened or streamlined. Rather than doing a comprehensive assessment of all performance and environmental components, the assessment can target only those that are relevant to the identified problem areas. If the COPM is done in addition to a battery of existing tests, or is seen simply as an add-on, then indeed it will take more time. If, however, the COPM guides the assessment process to include only those assessments relevant to the problem, then it should save time.

Another important consideration in the decision to use the COPM will be the service context. It is extremely challenging to practise from a client-centred approach in a system dominated and structured by a biomedical model. This is particularly true for those working in an acute hospital service where the emphasis is usually on rapid stabilisation and discharge. Here, the therapist's role may be quite targeted or specific, such as the prescription of a specific piece of equipment only, or the provision of a splint, and the domain of concern, a performance component or symptom relief. The COPM will not be appropriate in these circumstances as you are not really interested in the whole area of occupational performance. However, if the therapist's role is more concerned with discharge planning, the COPM can be a valuable tool to identify the issues that will be facing the client and the services that may be required. Community practice settings may lend themselves more easily to the use of the COPM in that the clients are often in their typical situations and may be currently experiencing some daily challenges, rather than trying to anticipate the challenges that may face them upon returning home. Services in the community may also allow more access to those in the client's environment who may be helpful in defining the direction for intervention, such as family, employers and teachers.

Although the COPM can present challenges in practice, these are really reflections of the challenges inherent in a client-centred approach to practice. Our experience and the results of several recent studies suggest that it is the philosophy and the skills of the therapist, rather than the types of clients or practice settings, that determine whether the COPM is used successfully.

CASE EXAMPLES

The case studies serve to illustrate the use of the COPM and some of the challenges inherent in its use. The examples include an individual respondent, a group of respondents and an organisation as respondent.

Community intervention

The COPM can also be used when occupational therapy intervention is provided for a group or a community or organisation. For example, a group of clients could have a shared occupational performance problem. The COPM could be

---

Case study: Margaret, an individual respondent

Margaret is a 79-year-old woman who lives in a hotel room in the city, having been evicted from her apartment. She was admitted to the assessment unit of the hospital for investigation of profound hypothyroidism and a rectal tumour. On admission, she was delusional, refused to take her medication, was unable to use her walker, unable to manage her personal hygiene or nutrition, and she was a heavy, hazardous smoker. There is no family support.

Although Margaret did not consider that she had any problems and that all she wanted to do was 'get out of here and go home', she did admit that she was not doing things she used to do. Some of these were:

* Self-care
  —'I can't use my walker, so I can't get to the bathroom.'
  —'I cannot manage to have a bath, even though I wash every day.'
  —'Keeping my clothes clean is a real problem.'
  —'I can't get around anywhere. Buses and taxis are too expensive.'
* Productivity
  —'I can't get out to shop.'

—'I just eat what there is, I'm not interested in cooking.'
—'I can't clean my place.'
* Leisure
  —'I wanted to travel to Cuba this year, but I don't have anyone to go with. All my family members have passed on.'
  —'I don't write letters any more. I can't hold a pen, or for that matter an idea in my head.'
  —'I used to be able to meditate, but can't do that now.'

The issues Margaret identified on the COPM, which she thought were important for her to be able to go home again, are shown in Table 10.1

The therapist worked with Margaret towards the most salient goal she had set for herself – going home. A variety of housing options were explored. In addition, the therapist focused on safety issues related to using the walker, smoking and cooking meals, and facilitated some increased insight into the client's behaviour. After an agreed upon period of occupational therapy, a reassessment was completed. The results are shown in Table 10.2.

Table 10.1 Initial COPM scores for Margaret

Problem	Performance	Satisfaction
Getting to the bathroom with the walker	2	1
Taking a bath	1	1
Cooking meals	1	1
Going out shopping	1	1
Total score	5/4 = 1.25	4/4 = 1.0

Table 10.2 Reassessment COPM scores for Margaret

Problem	Performance	Satisfaction
Getting to the bathroom with the walker	6	3
Taking a bath	4	5
Cooking meals	7	5
Going out shopping	3	2
Total score	20/4 = 5.0	15/4 = 3.75
Change in score	3.75	2.75

Case study: Jeremy; his parents and teachers

Jeremy Barker is a 13-year-old boy who has a history of learning difficulties and developmental coordination disorder. These problems have made school particularly challenging for him over the years. He has difficulty organising himself and his work, has limited attention and concentration, has difficulty completing written work, is fairly isolated from his peers, and receives 1 hour per day of special educational instruction. Jeremy is preparing to move on to secondary school. The occupational therapist is involved in planning for this transition with Jeremy, his parents and his teachers. She has interviewed Jeremy, his mother and his current homeroom teacher using the COPM. The results are shown in Table 10.3.

By interviewing the respondents separately, the therapist was able to understand the differing perspectives each person brought to the situation and the areas of concern that arose as they anticipated the transition to secondary school. This information was brought together in a conference and the differing priorities discussed. There was some congruence around the academic challenges facing Jeremy, but his priorities were, not surprisingly, more on the social aspects of school, whereas his mother and teacher were concerned about his academic progress. In the conference, the therapist worked with the individuals to negotiate some compromise and to help each person see how the areas of concern were interrelated. With initial agreement on the goals for intervention from each person, the chance of everyone working towards some common goals was enhanced. As well, when the time came for reassessment, the outcomes had been clearly articulated and were measured quickly and easily using the COPM.

Table 10.3 Initial COPM scores for each respondent

Respondent	Problem	Importance	Performance	Satisfaction
Jeremy	Making friends	10	2	1
	Playing sports	8	1	1
	Completing homework	7	3	4
Mother	Working independently	10	3	2
	Making friends	9	2	2
	Passing grades	9	4	2
Teacher	Coping with workload	10	2	1
	Independence	10	1	1
	Social skills	8	3	4

administered to the group to identify the occupational performance problems that should be the focus of intervention. If a community or organisation is the client, then the COPM interview still focuses on occupational performance, but from the organisation's perspective. A case example illustrates this.

The challenge in using the COPM in situations where the organisation is the client is to identify the best individual(s) to respond on behalf of the organisation. It is important that the COPM interview focuses on the performance problems from the organisational perspective, not from the perspective of a particular individual. In this way, the COPM can be used to gain a unique perspective on performance issues that are having an impact on the functioning of the organisation.

CONCLUSION

Outcome measures, based on a clearly defined model of practice, are essential to support quality occupational therapy service. Client-centred practice is a prevailing model of practice in occupational therapy and the COPM reflects many of the concepts inherent in the model. The COPM is an individualised outcome measure suitable for use with a wide variety of clients in any practice setting. It has demonstrated test–retest reliability, validity and responsiveness.

There are some challenges in integrating the COPM into occupational therapy practice. As it reflects a client-centred approach, the COPM is best suited for use within a client-centred rather than a professionally driven practice. Where clients have difficulty identifying their problems

Case study: An organisation as respondent

An occupational therapist is part of a task force for a local municipality. The purpose of the taskforce is to examine issues of accessibility to recreation services for persons with disabilities in that community. In this example, the municipality is the client. The municipality is represented by the taskforce, whose members are predominantly consumers, and also include staff from the recreation services department. Ultimate decisions about policy implementations are made by the local municipal council. The COPM was administered to the taskforce, made up of consumers and recreation services staff. The focus of the COPM interview was to describe how well the municipality provided accessibility to recreation programmes, and how satisfied the taskforce was with performance in the provision of recreation programmes. The issues identified that had led to difficulties in accessing and using recreation services included the following:

- training level of recreational staff
- physical accessibility of new municipal facilities
- affordable and accessible transportation
- availability of information regarding recreational programmes.

The results are shown in Table 10.4. Once these issues were identified, the task force (including the occupational therapist) performed an analysis to determine the specific causes of the problems identified. This information was collected through a review of legislated policies, information collected about recreational programmes currently available in the community, a survey of local recreational organisations, a survey of surrounding municipalities, site inspections of municipal recreational facilities, review of building codes, and community consultation of groups and individuals with disabilities. The information gathered from this analysis indicated reasons for the problems and suggested solutions. For example, consumers stated that municipal staff required more training with regard to disability issues and methods of inclusion and accommodation for participants with varying abilities. The recommendation was made that this training be provided on an ongoing basis and that resource people be identified who could assist municipal staff. In another problem area, it was identified that information about recreational programmes was not currently available in alternative forms such as large print, on cassette or in braille. It was recommended that alternative forms be used for programme information and that access information be included in all brochures about recreational programmes.

Table 10.4 COPM with organisation

Occupational performance problem	Performance	Satisfaction
Staff training	4	2
Access to facilities	6	5
Use of transportation	2	4
Access to information	2	2
Total score	14/4 = 3.5	13/4 = 3.25

in occupational performance, the therapist will need to adapt the assessment process to facilitate the full participation of the client and/or caregivers. The timing of the COPM, the fit with the health-delivery system and the practice location will all influence the ease with which the COPM can be used and the determination of its value.

ACKNOWLEDGEMENTS

The authors wish to acknowledge the contributions of Mary Law, Sue Baptiste and Hélène Polatajko, their co-authors of the Canadian Occupational Performance Measure.

REFERENCES

Baptiste S, Law M, Pollock N, Polatajko H, McColl M A, Carswell A 1993 The Canadian Occupational Performance Measure. World Federation of Occupational Therapy Bulletin 28:47–51

Bosch J 1995 The reliability and validity of the Canadian Occupational Performance Measure. Master's thesis, McMaster University, Hamilton, Ontario

Canadian Association of Occupational Therapists 1991 Occupational therapy guidelines for client-centred practice. CAOT Publications ACE, Toronto

Canadian Association of Occupational Therapists 1997 Enabling occupation: an occupational therapy perspective. CAOT Publications ACE, Ottawa

Department of National Health and Welfare & Canadian Association of Occupational Therapists 1983 Guidelines for the client-centred practice of occupational therapy. DNHW, Ottawa

Department of National Health and Welfare & Canadian Association of Occupational Therapists 1986 Intervention guidelines for the client-centred practice of occupational therapy. DNHW, Ottawa

Department of National Health and Welfare & Canadian Association of Occupational Therapists 1987 Toward outcome measures in occupational therapy. DNHW, Ottawa

Donabedian A 1976 Some basic issues in evaluating the quality of health care. In: American Nurse's Association (ed) Issues in evaluation research. American Nurses' Association, Kansas City, p 3

Donabedian A 1993 Quality in health care: whose responsibility is it? American College of Medical Quality 8(2):32–36

Ellenberg D B 1996 Outcomes research: the history, debate, and implications for the field of occupational therapy. American Journal of Occupational Therapy 50:436–441

Higgins C A 1997 Outcome measurement in home health. American Journal of Occupational Therapy 51:458–460

Law M, Cadman D, Rosenbaum P, DeMatteo C, Walter S, Russell D 1991 Neurodevelopmental therapy and upper extremity casting: results of a clinical trial. Developmental Medicine and Child Neurology 33:334–340

Law M, Baptiste S, Carswell A, McColl M A, Polatajko H, Pollock N 1994a The Canadian Occupational Performance Measure, 2nd edn. CAOT Publications ACE, Toronto.

Law M, Polatajko H, Pollock N, McColl M A, Carswell A, Baptiste S 1994b The Canadian Occupational Performance Measure: results of pilot testing. Canadian Journal of Occupational Therapy 61:191–197

McColl M A, Paterson M, Law M 1997 Validation of the COPM for community practice. Queen's University, Kingston, Ontario

Mahurin R K, Bettignies B H, Pirozzolo F J 1991 Structured Assessment of Independent Living Skills: preliminary report of a performance measure of functional abilities in dementia. Journal of Gerontology 46:58–66

Meyer A 1922 The philosophy of occupational therapy. Archives of Occupational Therapy 1:243–245.

Michalos A 1985 Satisfaction and happiness. Social Indicators Research 8:385–422.

Neistadt M 1995 Methods of assessing client's priorities: a survey of adult physical dysfunction settings. American Journal of Occupational Therapy 49:428–436

Northen J, Rust D, Nelson C, Watts J 1995 Involvement of adult rehabilitation patients in setting occupational therapy goals. American Journal of Occupational Therapy 49:214–220

Pollock N, Stewart D 1998 Occupational performance needs of school-aged children with physical disabilities in the community. Physical and Occupational Therapy in Pediatrics 18:55–68

Pollock N, Baptiste S, Law M, McColl MA, Opzoomer A, Polatajko H 1990 Occupational performance measures: a review based on the guidelines for client-centred practice. Canadian Journal of Occupational Therapy 57:82–87.

Rogers J C, Holm M B 1994 Accepting the challenge of outcome research: examining the effectiveness of occupational therapy practice. American Journal of Occupational Therapy 48:871–876

Sanford J, Law M, Swanson L, Guyatt G 1994 Assessing clinically important change in an outcome of rehabilitation in older adults. Conference of the American Society of Aging, San Francisco, California, Abstract no 811, p 100

Slagle E C 1934 Occupational therapy: recent methods and advances in the United States. Occupational Therapy and Rehabilitation 13:289–298

Steeden B 1994 Occupational therapy guidelines for client-centred practice and Canadian Occupational Performance Measure. British Journal of Occupational Therapy 57(1):23

Toomey M, Carswell A, Nicholson D 1995 The clinical utility of the Canadian Occupational Performance Measure. Canadian Journal of Occupational Therapy 62:242–249

Trombly C 1993 Anticipating the future: assessment of occupational function. American Journal of Occupational Therapy 47:253–257

Ware J E, Sherbourne C D 1992 The MOS 36-item short-form health survey (SF-36): conceptual framework and item selection. Medical Care 30:473–483

Wood-Dauphinee S, Opzoomer A, Williams J I, Marchand B B, Spitzer W O 1988 Assessment of global function: the Reintegration to Normal Living Index. Archives of Physical Medicine and Rehabilitation 69:583–590

Yerxa E J, Burnett-Beaulieu S, Stocking S, Azen S P 1988 Development of the Satisfaction with Performance Scaled Questionnaire. American Journal of Occupational Therapy 42:215–221

Index

Page numbers in bold type refer to tables and illustrations.